CARING FOR

How To Books for Family Reference

Arranging Insurance
Becoming a Father
Buying a Personal Computer
Caring for Someone at Home
Cash from Your Computer
Choosing a Nursing Home
Choosing a Package Holiday
Dealing with a Death in the Family
Having a Baby
Helping Your Child to Read
How to Apply to an Industrial
  Tribunal
How to be a Local Councillor
How to be an Effective School
  Governor
How to Claim State Benefits
How to Lose Weight & Keep Fit

How to Plan a Wedding
How to Raise Funds &
  Sponsorship
How to Run a Local Campaign
How to Run a Voluntary Group
How to Survive Divorce
How to Take Care of Your Heart
How to Use the Internet
Living Away From Home
Making a Complaint
Making a Wedding Speech
Managing Your Personal Finances
Successful Grandparenting
Successful Single Parenting
Taking in Students
Teaching Someone to Drive
Winning Consumer Competitions

Other titles in preparation

The How To Series now contains more than 200 titles in the following categories:

Business Basics
Family Reference
Jobs & Careers
Living & Working Abroad
Media Skills

Mind & Body
New Technology
Student Handbooks
Successful Writing
Travel

Please send for a free copy of the latest catalogue for full details (see back cover for address).

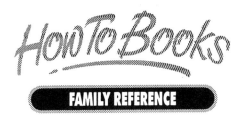

FAMILY REFERENCE

CARING FOR SOMEONE AT HOME

How to meet the needs of a
dependent person and their carer

Mary Webb

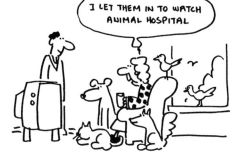

How To Books

By the same author in this series:

Choosing a Nursing Home

Cartoons by Mike Flanagan

British Library Cataloguing in Publication Data
A catalogue record for this book is available from the British Library.

© Copyright 1997 by Mary Webb.

First published in 1997 by How To Books Ltd, 3 Newtec Place,
Magdalen Road, Oxford OX4 1RE, United Kingdom.
Tel: (01865) 793806. Fax: (01865) 248780.

Note: The material contained in this book is set out in good faith for general
guidance and no liability can be accepted for loss or expense incurred as a
result of relying in particular circumstances on statements made in this book.
The law and regulations may be complex and liable to change, and readers
should check the current position with the relevant authorities before making
personal arrangements.

Produced for How To Books by Deer Park Productions.

Typeset by Concept Communications (Design & Print) Ltd, Crayford, Kent.
Printed and bound by Cromwell Press, Broughton Gifford, Melksham, Wiltshire.

Contents

List of Illustrations

Preface

There are thousands of people who have reason to be grateful to their carers. Carers work in hospitals, nursing and residential homes and in the community. Many people also, have dedicated their lives to caring for a relative or friend without counting the cost to themselves. This book is written for all carers but mainly for those caring for someone in their own home.

I would like to thank my husband Roy for his patience and support, Mrs Pat Reid RGN, the members of Scriptease and Hailsham Writing Group for their help and suggestions. The characters named in the case studies are fictitious as are the financial illustrations. Any similarity to other people or their circumstances is coincidental.

Finally I would like to dedicate this book to my caring daughters: Dawn Warboys RGN and Lyn Burgeman VN and all other carers with whom I have worked. Many of them have become my personal friends.

Mary Webb

1
Making Preparations

In this chapter the following will be discussed:

- considering the options

- customising the room

- resiting the fixtures

- choosing furniture

- keeping a homely atmosphere.

CONSIDERING THE OPTIONS

When there is a person in the household needing either supervisory or nursing care there are a number of options to be considered.

For example:

- care in a residential home
- care in a nursing home
- care at home.

Most people would prefer to be cared for at home if possible.

Being cared for at home

Being cared for at home has several advantages:

1. It stops sick relatives feeling they have been 'turned out' of their own home.

2. It helps to prevent elderly relatives becoming mentally confused.

3. It allows sick or disabled relatives to:

- stay in familiar surroundings
- be cared for by people they know
- to be involved in running their home, if they are able
- have a greater say in their care and treatment
- feel loved and wanted by family and friends.

Drawbacks

1. It's sometimes difficult to get extra help.

2. Your sick, disabled or elderly relative may feel bored or lonely.

3. Relatives can become 'difficult' with people they know and care for most.

ASSESSING ACCOMMODATION NEEDS

Long- or short-term care?
For a short-term illness such as a chest infection, you will probably be able to adapt the patient's bedroom to meet his or her needs. Light (unless light affects the eyes), airy and cheerful surroundings will help the patient to feel better. You may need extra space round the bed to give you easier access to the patient.

If your relative has a long-term or progressive illness such as Parkinson's disease or multiple sclerosis you may prefer to make permanent changes. This could involve choosing a more suitable room.

Choosing the new room
It's generally easier to care for an elderly or disabled person in a ground floor room. The choice however, depends on:

- what rooms are available

- your relative's mobility and dependency

- size and outlook of room

- toilet facilities

- ease for yourself, other carers and the general household.

CUSTOMISING THE ROOM

How you design the room will depend largely on your relative's mobility. As this may be the only room he or she will see for a long time try and make sure any changes are decided mutually.

It's always easier if the room can be cleared before alterations (if any) and redecoration are started. This isn't always possible due to the time factor or heavy furniture already in place.

Take into account what you can use in the room and what needs to be taken out. For example, if the room is currently the dining room the large dining table and dining chairs will not be needed. Nevertheless, a small drop-leaf or folding table may come in useful.

Deciding what to change

Make a list of what furniture and other essentials will be required in the room and what should be removed. The list in Figure 1 could be amended to suit your needs.

Furniture to be removed	*Furniture and other items required*
Dining table	Single bed
Dining room chairs	2 Easy chairs
Sideboard	Wardrobe
Heated trolley	Chest of drawers
	Bedside cabinet
	Over-bed table
	Commode chair

Fig. 1. A list of necessary and unnecessary furniture for the room.

RESITING FIXTURES

Check that fixtures, such as wall cupboards are placed so neither you or your relative will be caused injury. For example, it is inadvisable to place a cupboard over a bed in case something falls from it onto the person below. Have dangerous fixtures removed or put in a safer position if you still require them. Make sure that everything fixed to the walls and ceiling (smoke alarm and lights) is attached firmly and isn't likely to fall.

Thinking about power points

Consider your relative's needs. Are there sufficient electric sockets by the bed? These may be required for;

– electrically controlled bed

– ripple mattress

– bedside light

– radio

– electric blanket or pad

– other electrical items such as a fan or hairdryer.

Is there a power point in an appropriate place for the television? This needs to be located near the aerial point if there is one. Sockets may also be needed for electric heaters and cleaning equipment and these should be positioned in accessible places, not behind a wardrobe or under the bed. Consider the height – sometimes it's better to have them above a shelf or table-top if for example, you need an electric kettle in the room.

Siting a telephone point

If your relative is able to use and needs a phone you can either have a point put within reach of their bed or provide them with a cordless phone.

CHOOSING FURNITURE

Try to persuade your relative to choose the furniture that he or she would like to have in the room but be available to discuss what is needed. Bear in mind the following points when offering advice:

● Furniture needs to be practical as well as pleasant to look at.

● Allow space for storage of equipment and disposables *etc.*

● Chairs needs to be comfortable but not too large.

● Too much furniture in a small room gives a feeling of claustrophobia.

● Large furniture uses more space and leaves a smaller working area.

Making plans

It will help if you have some squared or graph paper. Either of these can be bought at a stationers. Graph paper is easier if you are using metric measurements (metres, centimetres and millimetres). Squared paper is easier if you are using linear measurements (yards, feet and inches). Measure the length, breadth and height of the chosen room. These measurements are useful for decorating purposes as well as planning the room. You can use either metres or feet and inches, as long as you use the same method all the time.

Draw the room to scale on your paper, for example one graph square to equal ten centimetres. Remember to draw in windows, doors and fixtures and mark down the position of gas, electric, phone and television aerial points.

Measure and jot down the size of the furniture that has to be fitted in. Take a look at the new room and try to picture the best positions for the necessary items.

Using your outline plan try to fit the furniture into the space where you want it to be. It helps if you cut out pieces of paper to the exact scale measurement of each item and fit them into the outline like a jigsaw puzzle.

● This will help you to decide the layout of the room.

● It will show where there is overcrowding.

● You will see where there is 'useable' space.

● Move the 'paper' furniture around in the plan until you find the best position – then try it out in the room.

Figures 2 and 3 illustrate room plans. Figure 2 uses graph paper and Figure 3 uses squared paper.

Making a list of furniture required

The following list could be amended to fit the needs of your relative.

– a suitable bed

– wardrobe or similar

– chest of drawers

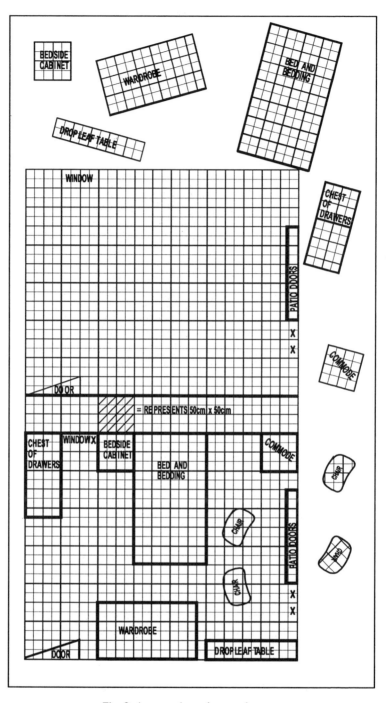

Fig. 2. A room plan using graph paper.
(Graph paper is usually 25 units to the square).

16

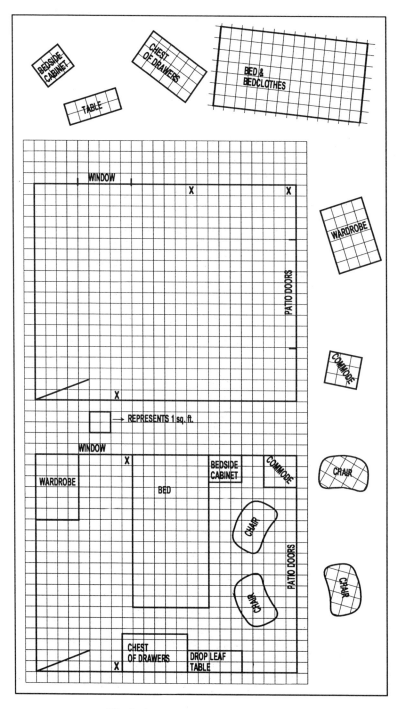

Fig. 3. A room plan using squared paper.

—   commode chair

—   bed table

—   comfortable chairs for relative and visitors

—   small table

—   bedside cabinet

—   cupboard for storage

—   space for walking aids and/or wheelchair

—   overhead light with dimmer switch, or bedside lamp.

Other items that might be needed:

—   bowl, face cloths, towels and toiletries (best kept in the bathroom)

—   back rest

—   bed cradle (to take the weight of bedding)

—   a bell or other means of calling for help

—   a book rest

—   special crockery and cutlery – often needed for 'stroke' victims.

Considering the bed

Depending on the needs and ability of your relative it is worth considering the most suitable type of bed. There are several different kinds of beds and mattresses on the market. The cost of these vary, and some will be beyond the pocket of the average person. However, if a particular type of bed is deemed by the hospital to be really necessary, they may be able to lend your relative one. Otherwise, it may be possible to get help with the cost. Such beds can usually be hired on a weekly basis and are collected by the firm when no longer required. Some of them are large and cumbersome and need more space than the average single bed.

Buying reconditioned
A few firms deal in reconditioned equipment. They sell beds that can be lowered or raised by using a pedal or have a built-in back rest or other gadgets – they will be less expensive than buying new. Extra accessories can usually be purchased separately. All reputable firms will guarantee their reconditioned equipment for a given period of time. Consider whether your relative needs or prefers a rigid base. This is particularly important if they suffer with back problems.

Looking at the mattress
You need to consider the mattress carefully. This is often sold separately and can range in price, governed by quality and type. If your relative is incontinent for example, consider a vinyl-covered mattress.

● They do not absorb spilt liquids.

● They are easier to keep clean.

● They can be washed over with disinfectant.

● After washing they can be dried quickly.

Although there are several different types and makes of mattresses the most well-known are probably the Spenco and the ripple mattress.

The Spenco type
The Spenco type of mattress goes on top of the ordinary mattress and is either made up of softly filled cells which fit into a special cover or is a one piece mattress. Some have a built-in waterproof for incontinent patients. A 'breathable' waterproof cover can be bought for those without this feature. The advantage of this type of mattress is that individual cells or the cover can be washed separately.

The ripple type of mattress
This type of mattress is powered by mains electricity, is made out of a vinyl type of material and is placed on top of the ordinary mattress. A ripple effect is caused by tubes, within the cover, inflating and deflating alternately with air pumped in by a compressor. This relieves pressure on vulnerable areas and helps prevent bed-sores developing.
     There should be nothing except a sheet between the mattress and the patient otherwise the effect is lost.
     You can still buy water beds but these are usually cumbersome and

are not always tolerated well by sick people. They are however, useful for the prevention of pressure sores.

Looking at bedding

It is more comfortable to have an underblanket between the mattress and bottom sheet, particularly if a vinyl mattress is being used. When using special mattresses however, such as a ripple mattress, this practice should be avoided.

● Always read the manufacturer's instructions.

● If in doubt get advice from the community nurse.

Using waterproof protection
Using a waterproof cover will protect a fabric mattress from spills or incontinence. These can be bought from most pharmacies. Although the use of an underblanket makes the bed more comfortable, it isn't practicle if your relative is incontinent. Try to compromise by using a flannelette bottom sheet.

Using duvets
Many modern establishments now use duvets to save time and effort in bed-making but some people still prefer to use blankets instead of, or to supplement their duvets. There are now waterproof duvets on the market for incontinent people. These are designed to allow perspiration to disperse but are not as comfortable for the sleeper as a fabric one. Coordinating duvet covers or bedspreads make the room look pleasing but make sure they are washable.

Have plenty of pillows available to support the patient while sitting up or being nursed on his or her side. Waterproof pillow protectors can be purchased but try to get the 'breathable' ones. They are expensive but much more comfortable.

Preventing mites
If your relative suffers from allergy to mites (which are microscopic creatures) it may be beneficial to have special mattress and pillow covers which can be obtained from the larger chemists. Sprays to prevent mites can be used to treat the mattress but get agreement from your relative's doctor first and be sure to follow the manufacturer's instructions.

Smoking
As people become more frail they tend to lose their memory and

coordination, often putting down or dropping their lighted cigarette on the bed rather than in an ash tray. If your relative smokes it would be safer to invest in flame retardant bed linen or limit his or her smoking to when you can unobtrusively supervise.

The lounge

Move furniture and television to meet your relative's needs when he or she has chosen where to sit. If the patient is blind be sure you explain any changes you have made to the layout of furniture in the room. Guide your relative through the new layout each time he or she walks about until more familiar with the changes.

The bathroom

Consider whether the toilet is the correct height. If not, toilet seat raisers of varying heights can be purchased. The toilet seat itself may be too hard and rigid for anyone frail. If this is the case, vinyl covered padded seats can now be obtained, at a reasonable cost, from most DIY stores. Foam padding, which can be bought quite cheaply from specialist shops and upholstery firms, can also be used to soften the seat.

The hand basin

If your relative is able to sit at the basin to wash themselves, consider whether it is necessary to have the height of the basin altered.

Using the bath

Ideally it is best if you can get right round the bath but this is not generally feasible in a private dwelling.

Assess the situation by considering the following questions:

- Can your relative get into the bath with your help?

- Do you need assistance to get your relative in and out of the bath?

- Is he or she light or heavy?

- Is a bath hoist required?

If you need assistance with bathing your relative ask the doctor to make a referral to social services or the community nurses. They may be able to offer help at home or make arrangements for your relative to be bathed at a local day care centre. Hoists and other equipment can be purchased either new or second hand. Make sure that second-hand equipment has been serviced and is in good working order before buying. If buying new, get the makers to fit and test the equipment before using it.

Floor covering
Many accidents, particularly amongst disabled, frail and elderly people are caused by floor covering.

Make sure:

- there are no loose or lifting floor tiles

- there is no chance that carpets or mats are likely to slip

- that there are no electric wires that could be tripped over

- that lino is not slippery (non-slip floor covering can be used)

- that spills are wiped up immediately.

Remember that some non-slip floor covering may still become slippery when wet.

KEEPING A HOMELY ATMOSPHERE

Many people, perhaps women particularly, like to decorate their homes with mementos, ornaments, flowers, pictures and photos. They turn living accommodation into a home and stamp it with their own individuality.

Bear this in mind when preparing the room for your relative.

- Ask them to choose pictures and photos.

- Let them decide what furniture they want.

- Try to prevent them from overcrowding the room.

- Flowers help to maintain a fresh, cheerful atmosphere.

CASE STUDIES

Introducing Eric and his sister, Alice

Eric is a 75-year-old widower. His wife passed away 15 years ago.

Although he was given bereavement counselling he has never got over his loss and still misses her. He suffered a stroke two years ago and since then has periods of confusion when he thinks Bunty, his wife, is still living in the house. He calls for her constantly.

Although Eric can walk quite well using a tripod he often forgets to turn off taps, and gas and electric appliances. Consequently, it is unsafe to leave him alone to care for himself.

He sometimes leaves the house to search for Bunty and generally gets lost. When he can't find her he becomes morose and depressed.

Eric is cared for by his younger sister Alice who lives with him. Alice works at home making knitted garments for a local firm. Pay is low but it gives her an interest and the chance to earn something of her own.

Alice keeps a diary, in which she jots down any significant happenings. She is going to share some of these with us.

Faith is terminally ill

Faith is 54 years of age. She found a lump in her breast two years ago which she tried to ignore. Her husband, who was a bully, would have physically abused her if she had gone to her doctor without his consent. He told her to forget it; that she was a hypochondriac and was only seeking attention.

It was not until an open sore developed that she decided to seek medical advice. She had experienced some pain but had controlled it by taking proprietary pain killers. Now the pain was much worse and had spread to her shoulderblade.

The open wound which she had treated with various creams kept weeping and she felt dirty. She washed herself constantly and splashed perfume over her skin. She wouldn't even meet her sister in case she thought she was not keeping herself clean.

Her doctor was appalled when he saw her and admitted her to hospital immediately. Faith asked him to notify her sister Anne rather than her husband. She was so distraught that he agreed to her wishes.

She wants to go home but can't face her husband and the responsibilities of married life any more. She is a very sick woman and her life expectancy is only a few weeks.

Introducing Grace

Grace suffers from Parkinson's disease. She is a 66-year-old, retired English and history teacher. She had been an excellent teacher and a kind, hard-working member of the staff who was liked and respected by both her pupils and colleagues. Grace worked in many countries and has friends living in Italy, America and Australia. She lost both parents when she was in her twenties and divorced her husband after five years of marriage because he was constantly unfaithful to her. She has no children. Grace has no financial problems and at present employs people to care for her during the day in addition to having a housekeeper and domestic staff. Relief staff have also been engaged.

Grace has some very good friends but her special friend is Sally who has been granted power of attorney.

Introducing Hannah

Hannah is 45 years of age. An accident 20 years ago fractured her spine leaving her with paraplegia (paralysis of the lower part of the body – below the site of the fracture). Hannah can do much for herself, including cooking and most household tasks. However, she relies on her husband Doug, to help her get up every morning and to go to bed at night. Community nurses visit daily to help her shower and check her pressure areas.

Hannah is cared for by Doug during the weekends, holidays and at night time. During the day her carers, Sarah aged 20 and Maureen aged 40, take it in turns to stay with her for two hours during the afternoons. A woman comes in daily to do most of the cleaning. Doug works as a store manager for the local council. Hannah writes in her diary every day and will be sharing some of her entries with us.

DISCUSSION POINTS

1. Does the room need redecorating?

2. Are there any pieces of equipment or furniture required?

3. Do any power or phone points need to be resited?

4. Do outside doors need alarms fitted?

5. Is the bed satisfactory or is a special bed required?

6. Is there sufficient bedding?

7. Would your patient prefer a duvet or blankets?

8. Does the bed linen need to be fire retardant?

2
Assessing Your Relative's Needs

In this chapter the following will be discussed:

- your relative's initial needs and feelings

- consulting the experts

- planning care

- changing needs

- keeping records.

LOOKING AT THE INITIAL NEEDS

People being nursed in their own home expect life to go on as it did before they became ill. Unfortunately, some illnesses can turn lives upside down by causing changes in outlook, ability and communication.

Making notes to help your relative

Make notes of your relative's physical needs. For example, can they:

- walk – with or without a walking aid   ———

- feed themselves   ———

- speak and swallow   ———

- dress themselves?   ———

   Is your relative incontinent:

- of urine   ———

- of faeces?   ———

If they are incontinent, is it because:

– They have a physical reason?   ———

– They do now know when they need to relieve themselves?   ———

– They are unable to get to the toilet in time?   ———

– They feel it draws attention to themselves?   ———

– They need toilet training?   ———

Thinking about pain
In order to help assess your relative's initial needs consider the following questions.

● Does your relative have any pain?

● If so, how severe is it?

● Is it mental or physical pain?

● What is causing the pain?

● How does pain affect them?

● Can the pain be controlled?

What is your relative feeling? Does he or she feel:

– anxious   ———

– apprehensive   ———

– angry   ———

– sad   ———

– happy?   ———

Some illnesses can change a person's attitude towards socialising. Many feel self-conscious about the resulting disabilities. Others look upon day care and luncheon clubs for the disabled and elderly as charity and 'wouldn't be seen dead' in such places. The acutely ill person generally feels too sick to cope with visitors, let alone other social activities.

Some people's religious outlook is changed by sickness and pain. A few will turn away from God because they feel their faith should have ensured immunity against illness. Many however, find strength and help from God and benefit from fellowship with visitors from the church. Writing down what you discover about your relative's needs will help you:

● to plan their care

● show new carers your relative's needs

● provide basic information for doctors and other professionals.

CONSULTING THE EXPERTS

Most people consult a doctor when they are ill. If you have been engaged professionally to look after a sick person, the doctor has probably seen your client fairly recently. On the other hand, you may be a relative who has taken on the task of caring. Your relative may have appeared reasonably well when you were persuaded to help, but is perhaps now becoming progressively worse. This is a time when you should ask the doctor to visit and re-assess the patient's health.

As the doctor may not have seen your relative for some time be prepared to provide full details of the illness. Here for example, are some of the ways in which illness can affect a person:

● insomnia (sleeplessness)

● tiredness

● poor appetite

● pain

● constant falls

● injury resulting from falls

● pale and/or abnormally sweaty skin

- excessive thirst

- frequent passing of urine

- frequent bouts of, or permanent confusion

- shakiness and tremors

- rash or sores

- apathy

- depression

- suicidal threats

- loss of coordination

- breathlessness

- paralysis of parts of the body (one side – hemiplegia)

- changes in temperature, pulse or respiration rate.

Be available when the doctor calls so that you can discuss any of these, or other problems. The doctor may refer your relative to hospital for investigation and treatment if necessary.

People with severe uncontrolled pain can be referred to a pain control clinic where their pain is assessed and treated. Patients with a terminal illness are sometimes referred to the nearest hospice for advice and management of their condition.

PLANNING CARE

Although you can make an initial assessment of your client's or rela- tive's immediate needs, it will take you a few days to make a more thorough assessment. If you are a close relative or friend you probably already know enough about the patient to make an accurate assessment of his or her needs. Bear in mind that relatives and friends are often quite different when you are nursing them every day to how they are when you only visit them at intervals.

Making a care plan

Figure 4 is a care plan which illustrates some of the immediate problems, and the action you might take to overcome them. If for example your relative is incontinent of urine it may be useful to keep a fluid chart (see Figure 5).

Date	Immediate problem	Action
6/6	Incontinent of urine	Try to find cause Regular 2 hourly toileting Encouragement Use of commode if this is easier Use of pads and pants Mattress protection Keep private parts clean and dry
	Frequency of passing urine	Keep a chart noting how much is passed each time Note how much fluid is being taken Discuss this with the doctor
	Frail and prone to pressure sores	Encourage to eat a well-balanced diet Use a Spenco or ripple mattress if available Nurse on alternate sides and back when they're in bed Give regular pressure area care

Fig. 4. An example of a care plan.

Date	Time	Fluid taken	Amount	Urine or other output	Amount
6/1	8am	Te	200ml	Urine (Incont.)	approx 250ml
	11	Coffee	200ml		
	12			Urine (Toilet)	300ml
		Total:		Total:	

Fig. 5. Example of a fluid chart.

As you get to know your relative you may realise that they have other problems you have not taken into account. Add these and the way you want to deal with them to the care plan.

CHANGING NEEDS

Review the care plan daily adding new problems and needs. For example: your relative may have an accident resulting in a leg injury. Initially it may need hospital treatment (*eg* stitching and dressing). You may be asked to keep your relative's leg raised for a few days and to ask the community nurse to redress the wound and remove the stitches in seven days. Enter this in the care plan on the day the accident happens and it will not be forgotten (see Figure 6).

Date	Problem	Action
8/6	Cut on shin. Sutured.	Keep leg raised to prevent swelling. Remove pressure bandage in 4hrs. Protect with non-adherent dressing and tubigrip. Sutures to be removed in 7 days.
	Pain from injury.	Get prescription from hospital or doctor for analgesia (pain killers) and dressings and tubigrip. Ask Doctor to arrange for the community nurse to visit.

Fig. 6. A care plan reflecting changing needs.

Prescription charges
Private patients pay for their private prescriptions and also the full cost of all the prescribed items. NHS prescription charges at the time of writing are £5.50 per prescribed item unless the patient is:

● aged 60 or over (man or woman)

● a child under 16

● between 16 and 18, in full time education

● diabetic or epileptic

- suffering from other selected chronic illnesses

- a war pensioner

- on income support.

Not all chronically sick people are exempt from charges but check with your pharmacist.

Prepayment certificates
If your relative is having three or more items prescribed regularly by their doctor it might be worth considering buying a prepayment certificate from your local pharmacy.

The current cost is £78.40 for a certificate lasting one year, or £28.50 for a certificate lasting four months. Bear in mind that these charges generally rise in April of each year.

Remembering facts

If you were asked in a months time how you *felt* today you would probably find it difficult to remember. If however, something of importance happened today you will probably be able to recall the date, the time and your feelings in a month's time. For example: if it is your daughter's wedding day today every moment will be etched on your mind.

It is however, more difficult to remember things when every day is little different from any other. Sometimes we *think* we remember but *do we*? Memory plays tricks and what we remember is not always accurate.

Doctors and consultants will ask you when a symptom first appeared or when your relative fell and injured him or herself. You may find that it's impossible to remember, because so much has happened since then!

KEEPING AND USING RECORDS

It's useful to keep a day-to-day record of your relative's health, sleep pattern, and anything else that you consider important. For example, a new drug may cause a reaction, such as nausea, loss of appetite, drowsiness, lethargy, a rash or something else. Any reaction should be noted and reported to the doctor who will treat the reaction, review and possibly change the medication. The doctor will need to know when the reaction started and how severe it was. If there has been a change of carers it may be difficult for them to find the information if it isn't written down.

Writing it down

Use an exercise book to write your notes in. Put your relatives name, date of birth, doctor's name and telephone number on the front cover.

Draw a right hand margin, wide enough for a signature. You should now have a right and a left hand margin.

Date	Patient care, observations, treatment and changes	Signature
	page 1	

Fig. 7. A sample record sheet.

If you are using loose sheets of paper to record information it will make it easier to keep them in order if you number the pages. Figure 7 is an example of a record sheet.

Use the left hand margin for the date. Use the main part for noting:

● your observations

● changes in your relatives physical condition

● psychological changes (mood swings, confusion *etc*)

● visits by consultants, doctors, care manager *etc*

● your relatives participation in social events

● changes in medication or treatment

- the giving and taking of medicines

- loss of appetite

- weight loss

- anything out of the ordinary concerning your relative's wellbeing.

Use the right hand margin for signatures of people making the notes. Biro should be used as it is more difficult to alter or erase.

Using the records
Your records are important for the following reasons:

1. They should show your relative's progress or deterioration.

2. They may be used by the doctor for assessment of your relative.

3. They will be used by other people caring for your relative in your absence.

4. They can be used in court if your relative dies unexpectedly in suspicious circumstances.

CASE STUDIES

Alice records Eric's fall in her diary

Saturday, 11 May
It was a bad day today, everything seems to have gone wrong. The day started off alright, Eric got up and dressed. It was sunny so we sat out in the garden. I only left him a minute while I went in to get our 'elevenses' and then it all happened. I heard a shout from the garden and looked out of the window to see Eric on the ground. I dashed out to him. He had a cut on the side of his head and blood was pouring down his face. He tried to move but yelled with the pain in his left hip. My neighbour had seen him fall from her bedroom window and had hurried down to see if she could help. She'd brought a cushion and a blanket with her because she knew we wouldn't be able to lift him ourselves.

We put the cushion under his head and covered him with the blanket to help prevent shock, she offered to stay with him while I went and phoned the ambulance.

The paramedic told me he thought that Eric had a broken femur and the cut was caused by hitting his head on a stone in the rockery. They thought Eric would be admitted to the ward at the hospital. They offered to take me but I told them I would drive in and take a few of his things in with me.

Eric had had an x-ray and was waiting to see the doctor again when I arrived. His head has been cleaned and dressed. I was surprised to see how frail he looked.

The doctor came to us after seeing the x-ray and said Eric would need an operation to have an artificial hip-joint fitted; he called it a prosthesis. The operation won't be done until tomorrow because they want to do some tests first.

They took him to the ward where they made him comfortable. He drifted off to sleep and I went to give the nurse all the personal information she needed.

Faith wants to go home

Diary entry: Friday, 19 April
I had a call from the hospital today; apparently my sister Faith is poorly. When I went to see her she looked ill but said she was feeling more comfortable now. She told me they had given her some stronger medicine to make the pain go away.

The sister told me that Faith had a very sore breast because she hadn't been to the doctor when she had first felt a lump there. She had apparently only gone to him because of the sore and the pain she had. But now it has been dressed. She told me that the nurse had put on soothing dressings and finished off with something that looked like a tea bag which she said was a 'charcoal dressing'.

The ward sister says that Faith wants to go home but she can't really cope. She has a terrible bully for a husband. He knocks her about when he doesn't get his own way. Faith is scared stiff of him. I expect he told her she shouldn't go to the doctor and that's why she didn't go. Sister also said that the tests they've done show that Faith's got secondary cancers in the spine and that she hasn't long to live. I've asked her to come and stay with me – I'll look after her! The ward sister said it would be hard work looking after Faith because she's so ill, but she thinks it's a good idea and will speak to the doctor about it.

Monday, 22 April
Before I got in to see Faith again her care manager (social worker) visited. She told her that she couldn't have 24-hour care like she did in

hospital if she decided to go home, but they would give her as much advice and help as possible. Faith apparently told the care manager that she had saved two thousand pounds for such an event and that perhaps it would be possible to employ somebody to help her. The ward sister telephoned and said Faith would be discharged as soon as I had the room ready. We agreed she would come in two days time.

Grace loses her appetite

Grace had always enjoyed her meals provided they were nicely served, with not too much on the plate. Mrs Green, her usual housekeeper, who had always cooked and served her meals had broken her arm and was off sick. The relief housekeeper overcooked the vegetables until they were unrecognisable. She had been told several times how to set a table and serve the food but still seemed incapable of carrying out the task properly. Grace tried to eat what she was given, but it wasn't easy. The food made her gag, but rather than complain she just gave up.

Grace was already slender but she began to lose weight and it soon became apparent that something was wrong. One of the carers decided to phone Grace's friend Sally and let her know what was happening.

Sally visited the next morning and was shocked to see how thin her friend had become in a few days. She stayed until lunch was served. It was awful. Brussels sprouts yellow with overcooking, tough meat, roughly mashed potatoes, floating in water and thick lumpy gravy that was congealing on the plate. The sweet was no better – a pie covered with lumpy custard and with pastry which looked and tasted like hardboard.

Sally went out to the kitchen to find the housekeeper tucking in to a ready-made frozen dinner! She told her to leave that afternoon and asked an agency to provide them with a more suitable housekeeper.

The new housekeeper produced appetising food but Grace still seemed to be having a problem. When this was reported to Sally she discovered that the dentures that Grace was wearing were the cause of the problem. Until her dentures were sorted out she was given soft, easy-to-swallow food supplemented with 'Complan'.

Hannah can't sleep

Diary: Monday, 20 May
I've always slept well but now I seem to be going through a phase where my mind appears to be working overtime. Thoughts and ideas churn round and round my brain until I feel as if I am going crazy.

I've tried all the usual things like counting sheep and my blessings but nothing seems to work.

Last night Doug heard me sigh and knew I was awake and so got up to find out what the matter was. When I told him I couldn't sleep he felt my skin and found that I was hot and sweaty and the sheets were damp with perspiration. Doug is so good to me. He never loses his patience and always gets up to me when I need him. He's looking tired these days – it worries me. I should hate anything to happen to him.

Doug brought in some tepid water and washed me, massaged my pressure areas and changed the sheets. Then he fetched me a warm cup of horlicks which I drunk through a straw while he cleared everything away. Afterwards he gave me a drink of water to clean my mouth. Just before he got back to bed he emptied my catheter bag in case its fullness was causing discomfort. I began to feel drowsy and fell asleep.

DISCUSSION POINTS

1. What do you feel are the immediate problems concerning your patient?

2. Which problem is causing the most concern at the present time?

3. What do you think will be the long-term outcome of your patient's illness?

4. How much can be spent on extra necessities?

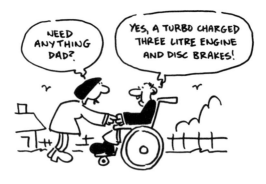

3
Organising Help

In this chapter the following will be discussed:

- making a start as a carer

- drawing up a rota

- filling in the gaps

- applying to Social Services

- hospice at home

- respite care.

MAKING A START AS A CARER

When you first start caring for your relative it will take a few days to get into a routine that suits both your relative and yourself. It should allow you sufficient time to give good care in an unhurried relaxed atmosphere.

Caring for a relative or friend

Many carers – particularly partners, family members (usually one) and close friends dedicate their lives to caring for a loved one. Often they are 'on duty' 24 hours a day, seven days a week. The carer becomes exhausted not only from the physical work but also from the responsibility of being on call night and day.

Carers often lose their friends because they are unable to leave the house unless they can get help for a couple of hours. Some are tied to their patient by moral blackmail. This makes them feel guilty when they go out even for essentials, such as food.

Carers also tend to lose interest in their hobbies and pastimes because it is too much effort for a tired brain and body to cope with. If you are one of these people make an effort to get some relief help even if it is only for a few hours a week.

Make time also to draw up a routine which will allow you some time to yourself each day, even if it is only half an hour. You will feel much more relaxed and more able to cope in times of stress.

Being employed as a carer

Some private families advertise for a companion/carer for a relative who needs looking after.

●   Make sure it is clear how many hours you are to be a companion and how many hours you are to be a carer.

●   Ensure you are being paid correctly for such a job.

●   Find out whether your client will need a full-time carer eventually.

●   Ask if this will affect your pay and working conditions.

Whether you are employed as a companion or as a carer, looking after someone in their own home, make sure you reach an agreement with your new employer regarding:

●   hours you will work

●   day duty, night duty or shifts

●   holiday and bank holiday entitlements

●   sick pay entitlements

●   salary

●   what arrangements will be made when you are off duty.

Usually your employer is a member of the family and you will be responsible to the family for the care you give. They may take over during your off-duty periods.

DRAWING UP A ROTA

If you need to employ a carer discuss with your family:

● the hours that your relative needs to be cared for

● how many carers will be needed each day

● facilities for the carers.

Some employed carers prefer to work fixed hours such as Monday to Friday 8am to 4pm whilst others are prepared to work more flexible hours. Bear this in mind when you are making out your rota. See Figure 8 for an example of staff rota.

Date	Day	Shift	Name of carer	Source	Comments
1/7	Mon	8–2	Debbie Meekin	Permanent	
1/7	Mon	2–8	Debbie Meekin		
1–2/7	Mon	Night	Josie Bloggs	Agency	
2/7	Tues	8–2	Anne Gilpin	Permanent	
2/7	Tues	2–8	Anne Gilpin		
2–3/7	Tues	Night	Josie Bloggs	Agency	
3/7	Wed	8–2	Anne Gilpin		
3/7	Wed	2–8	Anne Gilpin		
3–4/7	Wed	Night	Josie Bloggs	Agency	
4/7	Thurs	8–2	Betty Hart	Permanent	
4/7	Thurs	2–8	Betty Hart		
4–5/7	Thurs	Night	Cathy Linton	Permanent	
5/7	Fri	8–2	Betty Hart		
5/7	Fri	2–8	Anne Gilpin		
5–6/7	Fri	Night	Cathy Linton		
6/7	Sat	8–2	Anne Gilpin		
6/7	Sat	2–8	Anne Gilpin		
6–7/7	Sat	Night	Cathy Linton		
7/7	Sun	8–2	Betty Hart		
7/7	Sun	2–8	Helen Pusey	Daughter	
7–8/7	Sun	Night	Roger Price	Agency	

Fig. 8. Example of a staff rota.

FILLING IN THE GAPS

If you are a professional carer ask the family who they would like you to approach for more help. Some of them may be willing to sit with a sick relative for a few hours each day, even if they are not prepared to 'actively' care for them. If they are unable to help they may suggest other family members who could give a few hours, either on a regular basis or just occasionally.

Carers who are looking after relatives should ask the rest of the family for help either on a regular or casual basis. It may be possible to ask your relative's friends to help – but bear in mind they are of the same age group. You may find you have two people to care for instead of one!

● Discuss how many staff are needed.

● Ask social services if they can help.

● Check whether any members of the family can help.

● Try the volunteer bureau, the patient's friends, his or her church and any clubs he or she currently attends.

● As a last resort contact local nursing or care agencies.

Try to avoid using agency staff because:

● agency costs are high

● there is often a lack of continuity

● people who need care build a rapport with their own carers

● it's often difficult to get agency staff during school holidays.

If you do have to use agencies bear in mind the following:

● fees differ from agency to agency

● fees are higher for trained staff

● fees can be doubled for bank holidays

● higher rates are usually charged for weekends and night duty

- other charges may include:
  agency commission
  national insurance contributions
  travel allowance to and from your relative's home.

  If using agency staff you may be expected to provide:

(a) non-alcoholic beverages

(b) food – if the span of duty is longer than six hours

(c) coffee or tea breaks (approximately 15 minutes)

(d) meal breaks – if the span of duty is more than six hours

(e) cloakroom facilities.

APPLYING TO SOCIAL SERVICES

Approach your relative's **care manager**. The number of the local care manager's office can be obtained from your doctor's surgery. Every practice has been allocated a care manager who tries to sort out the social, welfare and care problems of their clients. The main groups of clients they assist are the elderly, the disabled, people with learning difficulties, chronically sick adults, those unable to care for themselves and those who are being cared for.

Your relative's care manager will do a 'needs' assessment as well as giving advice or practical assistance. If your relative is in hospital and ready for discharge they will give as much help as possible to ensure a smooth transfer back to their home.

Other sources of help

It is worth trying the local **volunteer bureau**. They sometimes have volunteers who will help out for a few hours a week. You must however, find out what the volunteer is willing or is allowed to do and also if they need to be insured whilst they are on your relative's premises. Church volunteers will sometimes sit with a patient for an hour or two particularly if your relative is a member of the church.

Finding a suitable routine

To keep harmony within the household choose a routine that's acceptable to your relative, the family, other staff and yourself. It will largely

Time	
7.30am	Toilet, wash and comb hair
8.00am	Breakfast and medication
9.30am	Toilet
11.00am	'Elevenses'
11.30am	Toilet
1.00pm	Lunch and medication (if any due)
1.30pm	Toilet
	Afternoon rest
3.30pm	Toilet, wash hands and face
5.30pm	Toilet, wash hands
6.00pm	Dinner/high tea, medication (if any)
7.30pm	Toilet, wash hands
9.00pm	Supper/hot milky drink
9.30pm	Toilet, wash hands, face and bottom, clean teeth. Remove and clean dentures, leave in soak overnight. Change into night clothes. Take your relative to bed and make them comfortable.
10.00pm	Give any medication that is due

This is the very basic routine. Other things such as baths and hair-dressing, leisure occupations, bed-making and manicures can be fitted in as convenient each day.

Fig. 9. Basis of a daily care routine.

depend on your relative's needs and wishes, and likes and dislikes. You will already have made a plan of the care to be given, now you need to decide the most appropriate times to carry out your planned care. Meal times are flexible, but bear in mind, that certain medicines and tablets must be given with food, whilst others should be given before, after or between meals according to instructions. Remember that if medications are to be fully effective they must be given regularly at the prescribed times. Most other daily tasks can be flexible, with the exception of toilet training.

If your relative has an afternoon rest you may be able to utilise this period as time for your own relaxation, even if you are unable to leave the house.

Planning the basics

Use a sheet of paper to jot down fixed times to do things, for instance: giving of medicines say 9am, 1pm, 5pm and 9pm.

It may be convenient to your relative to have meals at these times. If not give milk with the tablets.

You may need to take your relative to the toilet starting when they first wake up and then at two-hourly intervals, say 6.30am, 8.30am, 10.30am, 12.30pm, 2.30pm, 4.30pm, 6.30pm, 8.30pm and 10.30pm. (These times are only an example and would not suit all people.)

Cleanliness

Most people like to clean their teeth and wash before breakfast. This can be a bed-bath or just face, hands and bottom depending on whether your relative will be having a bath later.

These items then make up the basis of your routine and can be put into your daily plan first. Other tasks can be slotted in around them. See Figure 9 for an example of daily care routine.

HOSPICE AT HOME AND MACMILLAN NURSES

Doctors can refer patients terminally ill with cancer to the local hospice or the MacMillan nurses. Some hospices run their own service sending nurses out to visit and assess:

● the patient's wellbeing

● their pain level

● their drug regime

● any other problems that are related to their illness.

The nurses counsel their client and the family. They do not take on the actual nursing or caring of your relative while he or she is at home but they give advice and make recommendations to both the doctor and the carers regarding care and control of the patient's symptoms.

If they consider that they need to be admitted to the hospice for a few days, perhaps to alter their treatment, they will make the necessary arrangements.

ARRANGING RESPITE CARE

Respite care is very useful for anyone who is caring for a person single-handed.

- It gives the carer a much-needed break.

- It gives the carer a chance to go on holiday.

- Your relative's room can be 'spring-cleaned' while they are away.

- Your relative will get a change of scenery.

- There may be a possibility of physiotherapy in hospital.

Respite care can be arranged:

- privately with a local nursing home

- through social services

- possibly through recommendation by a MacMillan Nurse

- by recommendation to social services by your relative's doctor.

Your relative may be admitted to:

- a local nursing home

- a geriatric or rehabilitation ward in a local hospital

- a local hospice (for the terminally ill suffering from cancer)

- some other appropriate place.

Respite care is a short-term placement lasting one to four weeks. However, it may be of a longer or shorter period. Social services may be able to arrange two or three periods of respite care a year depending on the needs of the carer.

CASE STUDIES

Eric's sister Alice asks for an assessment in her own right

Diary entry: Wednesday, 15 May
I phoned Eric's care manager today. I told her that I never leave the house because he's not safe to be left. She asked me what I wanted and why had I phoned her.

I explained that I need some help so I can get out of the house occasionally. She didn't seem very interested but perhaps she was busy. They do seem to work hard, these care managers. Anyway, I asked if I could have an assessment in my own right like it says you can in the Carer's Act.

She replied that I couldn't have one until Eric was due for one. When I asked when that would be, she told me he should have an assessment no more than a year since his last one.

She was very surprised and apologetic when I told her that Eric hadn't even had his first assessment yet. She asked if she could come on Friday to do a 'carer's assessment'. So she's coming at 10.00am.

Helping choose helps Faith

Diary entry: Tuesday, 7 May
Faith is too ill to do much these days but she does appreciate flowers, particularly scented ones. She watched me from the lounge window when I went into the garden to cut some roses.

She's very conscious of any bad odours that hang around but doesn't always like the air freshener sprays I buy. When I went out today I noted the ones I thought she might like. When I got home I gave her the list asking her to choose.

She has decided to try a solid, long-lasting freshening block and two sprays, one for the bathroom and the other for general use. Although sprays give a pleasant odour instantly we both prefer having fresh flowers around the house. The nurses and visitors like them to.

Grace is feeling unwell

Grace was not her usual self on this particular day. It was an even greater effort to get up and dressed than it usually was. She said nothing to Jane, her carer, but Jane had noticed and decided to call the doctor if Grace got any worse.

She seemed a little better later on but had some discomfort in her lower back. Then she was incontinent of urine before she could get to the toilet. She was so upset and ashamed. Jane tried to comfort her but Grace remained distressed. Jane noticed that Grace's urine smelt offensive and thought the cause might be a urinary infection. She phoned the doctor who said he would visit and also asked for a sample of urine to be kept.

The doctor came quite quickly and agreed that Grace probably did have an infection. He prescribed antibiotics and suggested that extra drinks should be given. The urine sample that had been saved was sent for testing at the local hospital. Five days later Grace was feeling much better. The course of antibiotics had been completed and the doctor asked for another specimen of urine to go for testing to make sure the infection had cleared.

Hannah's husband, Doug, is tired

Diary entry: Tuesday, 11 June
Doug seems to fall asleep at odd times these days. He only has to sit down for a minute and he's asleep. I'm really quite worried about him. I don't know what I'd do if he became ill.

When Doug had gone off to work today I telephoned my care manager and asked him to visit. I hadn't met him before but he wasn't a bit like how I imagined a care manager would be. He was tall and thin, with a crew cut, an earring, an open-necked shirt and jeans – he looked more like a student. He was kind and understanding though and suggested that we should go away for a holiday together. I told him that Doug still wouldn't get a break because he'd still feel he'd have to look after me.

He then suggested that either I go into a nursing home for respite care or we go away for a holiday to a home that caters for the disabled. Anyway, he promised to look into the matter and suggested that in the meantime I should talk it over with Doug.

DISCUSSION POINTS

1. Will extra help be needed to care for your friend or relative?

2. Should somebody (other than the carer) liaise with social services?

3. If your relative is terminally ill should you ask for hospice care?

4. Will periods of respite care be required?

4
Using Available Services

In this chapter the following will be discussed:

● asking the doctor to make referrals

● helping the care manager to make the assessment

● managing incontinence

● buying, borrowing or renting appliances

● servicing of equipment.

ASKING THE DOCTOR TO MAKE REFERRALS

Discuss your relative's needs with the doctor; explain fully the reasons why you feel they should be referred.

The doctor may be reluctant or unable to refer your relative to consultants or other professionals because:

● he feels there isn't a need for a consultant's opinion

● your relative will not benefit from further treatment

● your relative has refused to seek a second opinion.

Any person who refuses to see a consultant or declines treatment cannot be forced, against their will, to accept what is offered. Sometimes parents, guardians or relatives make decisions regarding treatment for a patient. This might happen if the patient is a child or incapable of making their own decisions. It's possible that, in exceptional circumstances, these decisions can be overruled. The doctor would explain the reasons to you before taking action as it involves other doctors and one or more magistrate. Such measures are usually only taken in a life or death situation.

Case study

Shirley needs a blood transfusion
The car hurtled along at speed. The driver failed to see the small child crossing the road until the last minute. He slammed on his brakes but it was too late; he had hit her. She lay there, seemingly lifeless. A passer-by stopped and stayed with her while the driver phoned for an ambulance. As the child was taken to hospital he looked up and saw the notice 'Speed Kills!'.

Shirley, the little girl, had multiple injuries and had lost a lot of blood. She needed a blood transfusion. The police had traced the parents. They sat by her bedside but refused their consent for their child to be given blood.

They explained they were Jehovah's Witnesses and as such, they or their children were not allowed to have transfusions. The doctors spent a long time explaining the situation and how imperative it was that Shirley should have blood. The parents were adamant that no blood should be given to their child. They were willing that the child should die rather than receive the necessary transfusion.

The case was referred to the magistrates who overruled the parents. The transfusion was given and Shirley lived.

Asking for a referral
Ask for a referral to a:

● *consultant* if you are concerned about a medical complaint

● *community nurse* for nursing procedures (dressings, injections)

● *care managers* for home help, equipment, day care, respite care.

If your relative is referred to a consultant an appointment will be sent to him or her to attend the consultant's clinic, which is usually held at the local hospital. Your relative will need to get there in time for the appointment.

Transporting your relative
Whilst most elderly people find it difficult to travel by public transport there are many who find it impossible, usually because they are unable to walk the distance to the nearest bus stop or railway station. If you can't take your relative by car to the hospital ask the doctor's reception-ist to arrange some transport. Be sure to tell them whether a stretcher

will be needed, and whether someone will accompany your relative. There will be wheelchairs at the hospital for the use of patients.

Seeing the consultant

The consultant will ask to see your relative's current medication and may ask for various tests to be done, such as urine and blood tests. These will probably be done at the time and are to help the consultant make a diagnosis.

He may want to admit your relative for a few days of assessment and rehabilitation, particularly if he or she can't get about very easily. While your relative is in hospital:

1. He or she is likely to be given physiotherapy to help mobility.

2. He or she may be seen by the occupational therapist who will assess his or her ability to perform necessary day-to-day tasks. These are the things we all do for ourselves every day and take for granted. They include:

●   feeding oneself
●   washing and bathing
●   getting in and out of bed
●   sitting down and getting up from a chair
●   getting to and using the toilet – and getting back again
●   dressing and undressing.

The hospital will also assess whether your relative is able to:

●   make a hot drink for him or herself
●   and use electric and gas appliances safely.

Recommending changes

The **occupational therapist** may visit your relative's home before the time of discharge, and make any necessary recommendations. Safety is of prime importance both to the relative and other residents in the house. In addition to this they will consider ways of making things easier for your relative to live at home.

They will look at:

●   floor covering that might cause tripping

●   electrical appliances and the possible resiting of power points

- fires, electric, gas or solid fuel

- wheelchair access if appropriate

- toilet, bath, bedroom and lounge

- anything else that is appropriate to your relative.

Being discharged from hospital

The consultant may suggest that your relative is seen by a care manager before being discharged. This is to discuss his or her needs once at home again.

Any recommendations made by the occupational therapist concerning *eg* dangerous lino or carpets will be discussed. If your relative is agreeable, arrangements will be made for any recommendations to be carried out before returning home. Charges, if any, will have to be agreed with the care manager.

Asking for a wheelchair

You or your relative can ask the doctor or ward sister for a wheelchair if one is needed. Arrangements will then be made for your relative to be seen by the wheelchair department personnel. This is for an assessment to:

- find the most suitable wheelchair

- decide whether an electric wheelchair is needed

- assess what kind of chair your relative can cope with

- determine the size

- decide whether the wheelchair needs any modifications

- discuss attachments for example, tray, extended head-rest *etc.*

The chair may not be ready before your relative is transferred back home but it will be delivered as soon as it is ready.

HELPING THE CARE MANAGER MAKE ASSESSMENTS

When the care manager has been contacted he or she will visit to make an assessment. Ask if you can have a **'carer's needs assessment'** at the same time.

The care manager will take into account the amount of time and care:

- your relative needs

- you give as a carer

- given by other relatives and friends

- given by other organisations

- whether your relative needs to attend day care.

They will also need to know:

- full details of the care your relative needs

- the reasons why

- times when there is a shortfall of care due to lack of relief carers

- whether a trained nurse is necessary for dressings, injections or other treatments *etc* that you or your family are unable to do.

A financial assessment may also be carried out by the care manager at this interview. The information you give is confidential and will help to decide what help can be given.

MANAGING INCONTINENCE

If your relative is incontinent ask the care manager if he or she is eligible to have incontinence pads supplied through the health service and how to obtain them. Some areas supply them through the doctor's surgeries but other areas supply them through the community nursing services.

If you are obliged to buy pads try to buy them in bulk through a wholesaler as they will be cheaper than buying in small quantities. Make sure you give your relative's details and explain that he or she is paying for them. Incontinence products and nursing equipment are, at present, exempt from VAT when they are being used and paid for by the patient.

Disposing of used incontinence pads
Telephone your local council (refuse collection or environmental health

department) regarding the collection of used pads. Regulations tend to differ slightly throughout the country.

You will probably be required to put the pads into special sacks, tying and labelling them when full, before putting them out for collection. Most councils either charge for the provision of sacks and collect them free or make a monthly charge for the complete service.

Getting advice on incontinence and available products
Some firms selling incontinence products send out their own advisers. This service is free of charge but remember they will usually only advise on the products they sell and no others.

Finding unbiased advice
Unbiased advice on managing incontinence can be obtained by contacting the **incontinence adviser** employed by the Health Authority. Incontinence advisers are trained nurses who specialise in the subject. They do not prescribe, but they may suggest that you discuss the problem with the doctor. They will do this if they consider medication or catheterisation (passing a thin tube into the bladder so that the urine will flow into a collection bag) is appropriate. Incontinence advisers are normally based at one of the hospitals within your locality. For information on the best way to contact them telephone your:

● doctor's surgery

● the local hospital (geriatric ward)

● community nurse.

The adviser might visit your relative and may advise a 'toilet training' programme if it is thought that it may be of benefit. You will also be advised on the best type of pad, pants, sheaths (for men), urine collection bags, protective bedding and anything else related to this problem.

BORROWING, BUYING OR RENTING EQUIPMENT

If your relative needs a special piece of equipment, for instance a 'Mediscus' bed, there are three main ways in which you may be able to get it.

1. If a hospital consultant insists that special equipment or appliances are obtained for a patient's use before they are discharged it is

usually, but not always, hospital policy to install the item on **loan** at no charge to the patient. Ask your relative's care manager to make enquiries on their behalf.

There may be an agreement to read and sign and the item must be returned to the hospital when it's no longer required. Should your relative or representative contact the suppliers without official written authority from the hospital, he or she will become responsible for any payment that becomes due.

2. Your relative's representative can **rent** the necessary appliance from specialist leasing companies. They or your relative will be responsible for rental fees and possible maintenance and insurance.

    A contract will be given to your relative or his or her representative to read and sign, and return to the leasing company. Make sure you read the small print and if in doubt get it checked out by a solicitor.

    The contract should give information regarding:

    ● the weekly or monthly cost
    ● maintenance of the equipment
    ● emergency breakdowns and repairs
    ● how to return the equipment when it's no longer needed
    ● whether there will be charges for delivery or collecting
    ● any other charges, such as insurance.

    If the equipment is not insured by the leasing firm make sure it is covered through your own household contents insurance policy. When the equipment is delivered it should come with written instructions. After it is installed it should be tested on site, by the engineer or fitter. If instruction is not offered voluntarily, ask to be shown how to use the equipment. Most firms have a 'Help Line' in case of difficulty.

3. If you are considering **buying** equipment or appliances go to a reputable firm. The hospital should be able to give you any information you require.

    Smaller items such as bedpans and urinals can be obtained from some local chemists or shops specialising in goods for the disabled. Look in your local *Yellow Pages* for firms who specialise in equipment for the disabled. If they don't have exactly what you want in stock they may have an equivalent item or be able to get it for you. They generally have catalogues from which you can make a choice.

Don't forget to ask how long it takes to deliver. Hopefully this will be within days but sometimes it can take months! You may prefer to try other firms before committing yourself to a long wait.

Buying second-hand

Specialised goods are expensive and it might be worth trying firms that deal in reconditioned second-hand medical equipment. Most reputable firms allow you to visit their showrooms to view the goods before you purchase. They also guarantee their goods.

Remember that if medical equipment is being bought with the patient's money for his or her own use it is currently exempt from VAT.

SERVICING OF EQUIPMENT

Anything with mechanical or hydraulic parts, or run by electricity should be serviced regularly. Parts and wires can wear without the user being aware. Servicing needs to be carried out by a qualified person according to the manufacturer's instructions. If correct maintenance and testing is withheld it may invalidate the guarantee.

Should there be an accident involving your relative, or carers, the person responsible for the equipment may face prosecution if proper servicing has been neglected.

CASE STUDIES

Eric and Alice have an assessment of their needs

Diary entry: Friday, 17 May
Miss Smith, the care manager, came today. She wanted us to have a joint assessment of our needs but I wasn't happy about it. I knew that Eric didn't want anybody else in the house to help me and I didn't want her to think we could go on as we are; it's all too much. I asked her if I could have a private assessment and she agreed. She also apologised for not doing Eric's assessment before.

She started to ask Eric questions. He wasn't as confused as he often is and answered quite well. I was a bit worried Miss Smith would think he was a lot more able than he really is.

She asked him if he could walk and jotted down that he wasn't as mobile as he used to be. She wanted to know how much he could do for himself, what he felt he needed and lots of other things. Sometimes he could answer and other times he just looked at me and I answered for him. As the interview progressed his mind wandered and he became confused and difficult to manage. Then he started to call for Bunty. It took a while to settle him again. It was sad to see him like this in front of a stranger but I was quite pleased because it showed Miss Smith how difficult he could be.

Monday, 20 May
Miss Smith could see that Eric wasn't settled enough for me to have my own assessment on Friday so she came back this afternoon. She asked whether I wanted to go out to work and I told her that I needed to deliver my 'home' work. I also told her of my other needs and fears and she said she would look at the assessments and come back to me.

Faith is suffering a lot of pain

Diary entry: Tuesday, 14 May
I phoned the doctor today and asked for an urgent visit because Faith seemed to be in a lot of pain. He examined her, altered her drugs, then suggested that she should be referred to the **Hospice at Home** (MacMillan Nurses) who would advise the best way to control Faith's pain.

Because he told them it was urgent a MacMillan nurse called in early this afternoon. She looked at Faith's medication and then drew up a regime she thought would help. She phoned the doctor to discuss her proposals. When the doctor agreed she asked for new prescriptions to be written.

She told me that as soon as I had the drugs I was to phone her. She said she would come and set up a 'syringe driver' (a small machine that pumps the drugs into the body over a prolonged period at a set rate) to control Faith's pain.

The drugs arrived at 4.00 pm and I phoned the number the nurse had given to me. She arrived soon after and set up the syringe driver which she had brought with her.

She explained that this piece of equipment would remain the property of the hospice. It would however, stay with Faith until it was no longer needed. There would be no charge. The nurse said she would send somebody to check the equipment this evening and that she would come again tomorrow.

Grace needs a walking aid

Since Grace had developed the urinary infection she seemed to be more frail and unable to balance very well. Although she was feeling well again her walking has not improved. Her doctor sent her for some physiotherapy treatment. After several sessions however, she still lacked the ability to walk without some form of aid.

One day she was shown how to use a Zimmer frame which she managed very well. It steadied her and gave her confidence. She was sent home with one of the correct size and told to practise. She found that if a bag was attached to the front it was useful to carry things around in. The extra weight also helped to prevent her toppling backwards. Grace felt that she had regained some of her independence.

Hannah needs a hoist

Diary entry: Tuesday, 2 July
Like many other people I've put on extra weight over the last few years. I keep trying to diet but it hasn't made any difference. Anyway, the girls say I'm too heavy for them to get me in the bath any more.

Doug has phoned social services who have asked an occupational therapist to visit and advise.

When she came I showed her that there was no space for a hoist. She thought a powered bath chair might be feasible but would have to look into it. Near the bathroom there is a small boxroom full of household junk. She thought this room would be ideal to turn into a shower with a wheel-in shower tray accessed by a wheeled shower chair.

She asked me to discuss the idea with Doug, in the meantime she would contact social services regarding funding of such a project.

DISCUSSION POINTS

1. Would the family consider referral to a private consultant if there is a delay in obtaining a NHS appointment?

2. Who will go with your relative to any appointments?

3. Is there a need for a wheelchair? If so is an electric one required?

4. How safe are the premises for your relative and carers?

5
Satisfying Social Needs

In this chapter the following will be discussed:

- getting to know your relative's needs

- discovering your relative (or client)

- having visitors

- doing things in the home

- organising day care

- catering for spiritual needs.

GETTING TO KNOW YOUR RELATIVE'S NEEDS

The number and kinds of occupations your relative can pursue depend largely on their physical abilities and mental attitudes. It's easy to say that people *should* be stimulated into doing this and that if they *want* to do things. It's much more difficult however, if your relative:

- flatly refuses to be roused into doing activities

- is too apathetic to care

- is suffering from depression

- wishes only to sit in front of the television all day (and night)

- is wrapped in a world of their own that doesn't allow intruders.

It may take several 'talking' sessions before you can devise any ploys that will interest them. But you will gain personal satisfaction when you see your relative happily involved and enjoying him or herself.

When you talk to your relative try to discover:

- what (if anything) they would like to do

- whether there is anything they feel they 'have to do' before it's too late

- whether what they want to do is feasible

- hobbies they used to follow such as stamp collecting or crafts

- their past and current interests

- if they suffer any phobias that would prevent certain activities, for example agoraphobia (a fear of open spaces)

- spiritual feelings, problems and needs.

Religion can often be a sensitive subject and not easily discussed unless both parties are of the same religious persuasion. Nevertheless, it is important and can make a vast difference to your relative's psychological wellbeing and outlook, particularly if they have a terminal illness.

HAVING VISITORS

It's always a distraction when people come to visit. If the visitors are expected your relative will want to look his or her best and may take ages deciding on what to wear. Even if the patient is too sick to make the effort he or she will still appreciate having hands and face freshened, hair combed and the bed tidied. This applies to everybody but especially to those who were meticulous before they became infirm.

Timing

Visitors usually come with good intentions but often don't realise that a sick or elderly person tires easily. Fifteen minutes is a short time to a visitor but can seem like an age to a frail or sick person. Watch your relative closely for signs of stress. You may have to ask visitors to leave and come another day, or take them away for a while to give your relative a rest.

On the other hand, if they are well they will enjoy having visitors and there need be no restriction on the length of time they stay.

DOING THINGS IN THE HOME

There are several things you may be able to persuade your relative to take an interest in without leaving the house. Figure 10 is a list of possible indoor activities and Figure 11 suggests some outdoor activities.

Involving local organisations

Make enquiries at your library for the list of local organisations. Most libraries have a notice board especially for clubs and organisations to display their details and contacts. Note any that may be able to give assistance with any of the activities you and your relative have planned. Perhaps, for example, somebody from a gardening club may be willing to assist in helping with indoor and outdoor gardening. A member of the art club may like to advise and assist with projects connected with art. A member of a chess club may like to give your relative a game of chess occasionally.

Other organisations who may be able to send a member to help with activities are:

● *local senior schools* – approach the head teacher

● *scouts and guides* – approach the scout or guide leaders

● *your relative's church* – approach the vicar, pastor or equivalent.

ORGANISING DAY CARE

Day care will be organised by your relative's care manager, if it is considered to be beneficial. You will be told what days there are vacancies – your relative may have to wait a week or two for a vacancy to become available.

When the alotted day or days have been agreed you will be told what time the transport (usually a minibus) is likely to arrive. The minibus has to make several journeys to pick up clients and may not get to your relative exactly on time. It is very difficult for the driver to keep to a strict timetable so do not worry unless they are very late. If this does occur, telephone the centre and ask what has happened.

Happenings at day care

Your relative will need to take some money to the day-care centre to pay for lunch. This is usually a minimal sum, but apart from helping to defray the cost it gives your relative a small measure of independence.

Activity	Equipment needed
TV, Radio, records, tapes	Television, music centre or equivalent
Playing board games	Games compendium or equivalent
Cards	Pack of cards: large print if possible
Jigsaw puzzles	Various puzzles – borrow from library
Art (simple or advanced)	Water or oil paints, brushes, canvasses or equivalent, cleaning agents, protection for furniture and relative somewhere to hang pictures to dry
Collage	Any scraps of materials, dried pulses, sequins, buttons, braids *etc*, glue, strong paper, glue brush, protection for furniture and relative
Reading	Books from library
Talking books/newspaper	Primarily for the blind person
Crafts	Sewing materials are usually required, in addition to any specific items needed for the chosen craft
Cake making	Apron, ingredients, supervision
Cake decoration	Apron, ingredients, supervision

Fig.10. A list of indoor activities.

Activity	Equipment needed
Outdoor gardening	Raised flower beds helpful, gardening plants *etc*, protective clothing and shoes, fine weather
Greenhouse gardening	greenhouse
Shopping	Wheelchair or other aids, transport
Going to 'day care'	Transport, wheelchair if necessary
Outings	Transport, escort, extra pads if used
Out for a walk	Wheelchair, adequate clothing
Trips to gardens	Transport, wheelchair if necessary
Trips to theatre	Booked seats (wheelchairs not always accepted)

Fig. 11. Some ideas for outdoor activities.

You will need to send any necessary lunch-time medicines for your relative to take and ensure that the staff are aware of what time the medication is to be taken.

At the day centre, coffee, lunch and afternoon tea are provided. In between there is time to chat, do movement to music (gentle exercise) Bingo and other things that are on the scheduled programme. If you have difficulty bathing your relative ask if they could do this for you. If they agree, send clean clothing for your relative to put on afterwards. Sometimes physiotherapy can be given if requested by the doctor.

Some heads of day care arrange outings, parties and entertainments for their clients but there may be a small charge for outings. Clients are usually taken home about 4.00pm.

You will need to check the following:

● approximate time transport will arrive for your relative

● approximate time he or she will arrive home

● what day(s) he or she will go to day care

● how much money will be needed each day

● which day a bath will be provided (if you have arranged this)

● that they know your relative takes medication at lunch time.

Always notify the day centre if your relative is ill and can't attend. This will give them the chance to cancel the transport, providing you are able to tell them early enough.

If there are any problems always go and discuss them with the day-care staff. *Remember*, day-care staff cannot sort out a problem unless they have been told that there is one.

CATERING FOR SPIRITUAL NEEDS

It can be difficult to assess the spiritual needs of the person for whom you are caring.

It may be something you can establish during one of your 'talking' or discussion sessions. Check which denomination your relative belongs to. Contact the chosen church and arrange for the vicar, pastor, rabbi, priest or other leader to visit if this is what your relative wishes.

He or she may also appreciate visits from other church members and to be kept informed about church activities.

Often people who refuse spiritual help change their minds as the end of their life approaches. They begin to wonder what lies ahead of them; they may worry about death and beyond. Many unbelievers feel afraid to die, yet afraid to ask for help.

If you feel your relative needs spiritual comfort or help, ask his or her permission to send for an appropriate person or discuss the situation with the family.

CASE STUDIES

Eric goes to day care

Diary entry: Tuesday, 21 May
Miss Smith visited again today, she had been busy on our behalf. She said Eric could go to day care two days a week. On those days she would arrange for a carer to come and get him up and ready and stay with him until he was collected. She was also able, if I wanted to go out for the day, to get a carer to look after him until I returned. I feel very happy that she has managed to assist in this way. Not only can I

get out sometimes but it will also give me a chance to catch up on the housework.

I accepted her offer. Eric will start going to day care next week on Tuesdays and Thursdays.

Faith needs spiritual comfort

Diary entry: Thursday, 16 May
Faith has been a member of the Pentecostal Church for years, although she hasn't been active for some time. Now that she knows she hasn't long to live she feels the need to talk to the Pastor.

I phoned and spoke to him regarding my sister this afternoon. He has promised to visit her tomorrow.

Friday, 17 May
The Pastor called today. He talked to Faith and read from the Bible and prayed with her. She felt better and at peace. He asked if she would like other members of the church to visit. When she said she would, he offered to make the arrangements.

Monday, 20 May
A package arrived today brought by one of the members – it was a recording of yesterdays services. Faith was delighted. Her husband has kept away so far – fortunately.

Grace needs new clothing

Grace's carers were concerned because her underwear and nightdresses were worn and tatty. They also noticed that she hadn't any winter dresses either. They decided to speak to Sally and see if she could get Grace some new clothing.

Sally asked the carers to make a list of everything that she needed and to put the things to be replaced in a pile for her to look at. She then went out and priced everything so that she could put an estimated cost to the solicitor and get sufficient money from the estate to buy the goods.

The solicitor gave permission for the clothing to be purchased but needed all the receipts.

Sally bought all things with the understanding they could be returned or exchanged if they were unsuitable. Grace and the carers were delighted with her new dresses and underwear.

Sally kept all the receipts and sent them to the solicitor as he had requested.

Hannah goes on holiday

Diary entry: Monday, 8 July
My care manager has arranged for me to go into a nursing home for two weeks respite care. One of my friends lives 20 miles from us, on the Kent coast. She has recommended a nursing home near to where she lives. She will be able to drive me to the home and also take me out to places of interest. Doug is letting her use our specially adapted car. He's decided to fly to Jersey for a few days, arriving home the day before me.

I'm really busy now, making lists of what I want to take and what Doug needs for his holiday. He got the cases down yesterday and I'm gradually filling them with holiday things.

I phoned the surgery today to renew my prescriptions for more catheters and urine bags so I will have enough to take with me.

DISCUSSION POINTS

● What activities do you think your relative would be interested in?

● How will outings and craft materials be funded?

● Some religions have special customs for when one of their followers dies. Discuss whether this applies to your relative.

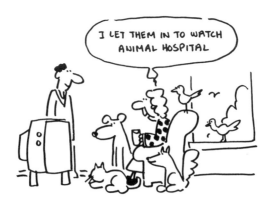

6
Considering Your Responsibilities

In this chapter the following will be discussed:

- domestic duties

- keeping the house fresh

- involving your relative

- providing a nourishing diet

- working with other staff.

LOOKING AT DOMESTIC DUTIES

Some carers, particularly family members, may find themselves responsible for keeping the home clean and tidy. This is in addition to caring for their sick relative. Discuss with the rest of the family the amount of housework you are expected to do. If you are to be employed as a carer make sure this point is discussed clearly at your interview. (See Chapter 3 page 38).

The main carer should assess the amount of domestic work that has to be done each day. Don't forget to include everything that might be termed as domestic work such as:

- dusting, hoovering, sweeping and washing floors

- cleaning windows, washing down paintwork

- personal and household laundering

- washing, drying and putting away eating and cooking utensils

- your relative's personal and household shopping

- preparing and cooking meals *etc.*

Estimate how many hours you will spend doing household tasks. While you're doing domestic work you can't be with your relative in a caring capacity.

If you find there is more domestic work that you can feasibly cope with, discuss the possibility of employing domestic staff with:

- your relative (if possible)

- the rest of the family

- the person who has power of attorney

- your employer.

Make sure you give a full explanation of why extra domestic help is necessary. You may find it useful to work out a routine. Make notes of the time the various jobs take and how your sick relative coped when you were doing them. Take these notes with you when you ask for extra help, they will support your case.

When you are trying out various routines remember that you will have to show employees how you want the work to be done. Make sure you choose a routine that will work for:

- your relative

- other carers

- newly appointed employees

- housekeeper/domestic staff.

KEEPING THE HOUSE FRESH

A house that smells fresh is:

- pleasant for your relative

- is pleasing for visitors

- agreeable to yourself and other staff.

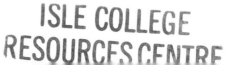

It's easy to become insensitive to odours around you if you live and work in the same place. Explosive smells such as that of faecal incontinence is easy to detect, but the smell of uncontrolled urinary incontinence builds up and can go unnoticed by people living with it.

If you are not careful urine can spill and leak into furnishings and carpets. Although you may wipe spills up quickly a smell of stale urine can soon permeate the house. Unfortunately, a carer, working or living in this kind of situation can find that they don't notice the smell because they have got used to it. However, visitors coming into the house will. Some are discouraged from visiting by an unpleasant odour.

Coping with unpleasant smells

Check that your relative does not suffer from allergies to sprays *etc*. If the odours are caused by incontinence try to start a toilet training programme. See Chapter 3 page 43.

The following tips will help prevent long-term unpleasant odours:

● Change wet or soiled clothing, bed linen and pads immediately.

● Put soiled or wet clothing or bed linen into plastic linen bins.

● Never put soiled or wet linen or used pads on the floor or furniture.

● Dispose of used pads into plastic bags and seal them.

● Wash or soak soiled linen as soon as is practical.

● Always wipe up spills immediately.

● Wash or use appropriate cleaners for furniture and carpets.

● Treat the area with an appropriate odour absorber.

● Use aerosol sprays, if they can be tolerated.

● Use solid deodorising blocks.

● Use, (in extreme cases) colostomy deodorising fluid.

Because you may not be able to detect odours yourself doesn't mean that there isn't one. Get a friend to tell you if the house smells pleasant or not.

Dishes of potpourri or sweet scented flowers such as roses, freesias or lavender look inviting and help to mask any lingering traces of unpleasant whiffs. You can also try using scented candles but make sure they are not a fire risk.

INVOLVING YOUR RELATIVE

Providing that your relative is able, and willing, he or she may enjoy helping with minor, day-to-day household tasks: choosing the fragrances or sprays you use for conditioning the air or arranging the flowers.

Other appropriate jobs may include:

- cleaning the silver

- setting the table for meals

- folding serviettes

- helping to plan the menu

- preparing vegetables *eg* shelling peas.

These are just a few things that you may find your relative would like to help with. You can add other little jobs to the list.

PROVIDING A NOURISHING DIET

A good diet must provide everything necessary to maintain or improve health. It should be composed of a variety of food that:

- is served attractively

- looks and smells appetising

- tastes delicious

- is easy to eat and digest.

It's no use giving your relative tough meat even if it fulfills all the other criteria. They won't be able to chew it. In fact it may cause them to choke. Even if they can swallow it they will probably suffer from indigestion afterwards!

Planning menus

When planning menus take into account:

● your relative's likes and dislikes

● any food allergies that he or she may suffer from

● whether he or she has dentures

● whether the dentures fit properly

● whether he or she is used to a main meal at midday or in the evening.

There may also be some dietary requirements for controlling a medical condition. For example:

– low salt or salt free diet
– low fat or fat free diet
– diabetic diet
– reducing diet for obesity
– liquid or semi-solid diets.

Think about the main nutrients of a nourishing diet:

1. protein

2. carbohydrates

3. fat

4. minerals for example: iron

5. vitamins for example: A, B, C, D, E, K

6. trace elements for example: manganese, fluorine, copper *etc.*

7. calcium

8. at least five glasses of water daily which can be made up of herbal tea, mineral water, fruit juices, tea and coffee (made with water). In hot weather your relative might like to try iced tea or coffee.

See Figure 12 which is a nutrition chart and will tell you where nutrients and vitamins are found and what they are needed for.

Nutrient	Found in these foods	Required for
Protein	Meat, fish, eggs, milk, cheese, peas, beans, lentils, cereals, root vegetables.	Strong bones, replacing exhausted cells, repair of muscle tissue growth
Carbohydrates	All products containing sugar *ie* sweets, jam. All products made with flour. Cereals. Some root vegetables. Potatoes.	Energy
Fats	Butter, lard, all oils, margarine and cooking fat, dripping, cream, cheese, egg yolk, salad cream, fish oils.	Energy
Water	Fruit and vegetables, almost all other foods.	Crucial for body cells and almost all bodily functions.
Vitamins		
A	Fish liver oils, fats, carrots, tomatoes, dark green leafy vegetables, dairy products.	Resistance to infection. Growth. Deficiency may lead to night blindness and eye diseases.
B Complex	Nuts, liver, yeast, wholemeal bread, oats, dairy products, kidney.	Maintains red blood corpuscles and nerve cells.
C	Most fruit and vegetables.	Helps with healing wounds, growth and bone development.
D	Eggs, sardines, herrings, dairy products.	Essential for the absorption of calcium.
E	Soya beans, wheatgerm, egg yolk, cereals, meat and fish, nuts, green leafy vegetables.	Helps to prevent cell degeneration.
K	Polyunsaturated fats, leafy green vegetables, cereals, milk, eggs.	Needed for normal blood clotting
Salt	Many kinds of foods.	Essential for maintaining the body's water balance, regulates activity of muscles and nerves.
Trace elements Copper, zinc *etc.*	Many kinds of food.	Needed for normal metabolism.
Calcium	Milk, cheese.	Necessary for bones and teeth.
Iron	Liver, eggs, cereals, green vegetables, wholemeal bread, pulses.	Prevents iron deficiency, anaemia. (Vitamin C helps absorption.)

Fig. 12. A nutrition chart.

Breakfast

Grapefruit or fresh fruit juice
Porridge or high fibre cereal
Toast (wholemeal if possible)
Low fat spread
Marmalade, jam or honey
Tea or coffee

Lunch

Steamed fish with parsley sauce
Boiled potatoes
Peas and carrots
Apple crumble and custard
Tea or coffee

High tea

Soup
Poached egg on wholemeal toast
Cake
Fresh fruit
Tea or coffee

Supper

Milky drink (Horlicks, malted milk)
Sweet biscuits or cream crackers

Fig. 13. Sample menu for an elderly person on a normal diet.

Where possible use foods with a high fibre content, for example: beans and pulses, brown rice, pasta and wholemeal bread. Fibre in the diet stimulates digestion and helps to prevent constipation and cancer of the digestive system.

Figure 13 provides a sample menu for an elderly person on a normal diet.

Coping with special diets

There are several different diets that can be ordered by the doctor. They are given to help your relative recover or to prevent his or her condition deteriorating.

If you need to know how to cope with any such prescribed diet ask to see a dietician. There will probably be an appropriate leaflet at the surgery which may help you plan attractive nourishing meals for your relative whilst avoiding any prohibited ingredients.

Being restricted to a fluid diet

If your relative can only have a **fluid diet** they should have about 20 cups of fluid each 24-hour period. Check this amount with the doctor, particularly if your relative is suffering from fluid retention or heart problems.

At least half the amount to be given should be of a milk-based drink. Not everybody likes plain milk but it can be made into a:

● milk-shake with flavouring and ice cream.

● soup (no lumps)

● fortified drink – flavoured or plain Complan or similar substance. Other drinks can include Hycal (a fortified sweet drink on prescription) Bovril, fruit juice or squash.

Keeping to a light diet

A **light diet** would be made up of chicken or turkey breast (no skin), fish, egg, bread and butter plus small amount of vegetables.

Going on a diet

Nobody should be given a diet for **obesity** unless the doctor has examined them and has approved the diet to be given. If the doctor feels that such a diet is necessary he will refer your relative to the dietician. He or she will then be interviewed and weighed, if possible, before being given a tailor-made diet. The dietician will want to check your relative's progress at regular intervals.

Managing diabetic diets
People suffering from **diabetes** must visit the dietician who will work out their dietary needs and discuss their diet with them and the person caring for them. Most diabetics can eat a healthy normal diet which should be fully understood by the patient and the carer.

You will need to carry out regular urine tests for sugar and probably test your relative's blood for sugar as well. These tests are quite simple to do and you will be shown the correct way of doing them by the community nurse or the practice nurse at the surgery.

If your relative is newly dependant on insulin injections these may be given and monitored by the community nurse until your relative is able to do them independently. Discuss with the doctor, the community nurse or the diabetic nurse specialist the best way to administer the dose. It is possible that your relative could be prescribed a special 'pen' that will help.

Regular check-ups at the diabetic clinic, optician and chiropodist are essential.

Note: People suffering from diabetes are exempt from prescription charges, whatever their age.

Helping a blind person retain independence at meal times
If your relative is blind he or she will require special consideration at meal times, whilst at the same time being allowed to retain his or her independence.

1. Explain now many courses there are and what the menu is.

2. Tell him or her to think of the plate as a clock face (see Figure 14).

3. Explain where the different kinds of food are in relation to the hours.

4. Make sure he or she has all the utensils for eating.

5. Explain where the condiments are in relation to their plate.

6. Tell him or her where to find the glass and what's in it.

7. Make sure he or she knows where the serviette is.

8. Be close at hand in case help is needed.

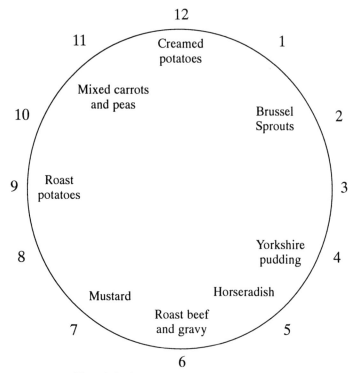

Fig. 14. Setting out the plate like a clock face.

WORKING WITH OTHER STAFF

This can be quite a complex problem because of differing personalities between the staff. Occasionally two people either instantly like or dislike each other. Fortunately however, such instant judgements are seldom made and relationships tend to build over a period of time. Nevertheless, sometimes two people are unable to work with each other. If this does happen, try to get the people concerned to work at different times.

Dealing with staff already in post

Whether you are the caring relative or an employed carer and new to the household you may find there is some resentment and fear shown by other staff especially those who have been in post for a long period of time. Resentment may occur because anyone new is seen as an usurper. Existing staff may also feel threatened by the arrival of someone new. Their fears may be based on some of the following reasons:

1. You may change all the established routines. You may be told: 'It's been done this way for as long as I can remember. I don't see why we should change now.' The method they're using may be, in your opinion, unhygienic or unsafe; but it's sometimes difficult even to get them to consider a different approach.

2. You may need waiting on hand and foot, causing them much more work.

3. You may come between them and their elderly or disabled employer. Many old retainers are more than just a housekeeper or a domestic. They have, in the past, become a trusted friend to their employer and have given the care that you, as the carer, have now taken on.

4. You may eventually drive them out of their job. They may feel they are no longer needed. Long-term residential employees may not have another home and visualise themselves homeless and penniless. Reassurance, tact and patience are required to reach a happier situation.

Don't be afraid to ask for their help. Try to involve any existing staff in caring for your relative. Offer them opportunities to sit and talk to your relative so that the friendship can continue. This gesture will almost certainly be appreciated.

Remember you are part of a well-established team working together for the happiness, comfort and wellbeing of your relative.

Employing new staff
You may or may not be responsible for engaging new staff. That will be up to the family or your employer. However, if this is your responsibility be sure you:

● advertise the post appropriately

● ask for the applicant's CV

● arrange interviews

● make notes, in case you forget salient points

● compile a 'short-list' (if you have several applicants to interview)

● arrange a second interview if required

- give applicants full details of the post

- request the successful applicant's P45.

- remember it is illegal to pay 'cash in hand' without declaring your employee's earnings to HM Inspector of Taxes.

- tell any self-employed persons who work for you that they will be responsible for paying their own tax and National Insurance Contributions (NIC). To protect yourself from any future tax problems you should inform the HM inspector of Taxes.

Figure 15 outlines the procedure for employing new staff. Figure 16 is an interview sheet with examples of some questions to ask the applicant.

Welcoming new staff

Their first day
Be sure to greet the new member of staff in a friendly manner. Remember they may be suffering from first day nerves.

On the first day they will need to be shown around and instructed in their duties. Make sure you know what is to be done and be prepared to show them how. Demonstrate how mechanical aids work, *eg* the washing machine. It may save money being spent on repairs!

Always remember to thank them when they have finished. Make sure both you and they know when they are to come again.

CASE STUDIES

Helping in the garden

Diary entry: Wednesday, 22 May
Eric has changed, he seems to have lost interest in everything since his fall. At least he doesn't go wandering out of the house now and getting himself lost.

He used to be a keen gardener so I thought I would try and get him to plant some seeds today. At first, all he wanted to do was sit down so I let him sit in a comfortable chair and put a table in front of him. I put some seeds, some trays and compost on it, then I started. He began to help, heaping compost into trays and smoothing it out.

Then he pushed the table away and walked to the shed. I was so surprised when he came out clutching some plant markers and a pencil. He came back to his chair and tried to write the names on the marker but that was too much for him. He gave them to me to do. As we had filled the seed trays I put them on the ground then gave him a half filled watering can. He kept pointing to the spout and I realised he wanted the rose. Once that was fitted he watered them and I put the trays in the greenhouse. We finished up sewing some mustard and cress. I thought he would enjoy seeing how quickly it grew and eating it when it was ready.

Eric enjoyed the afternoon – he hadn't called for Bunty at all whilst he was helping in the garden.

Faith's sister, Anne, employs part-time help

Diary entry: Wednesday, 22 May
I put adverts in the local paper and the Job Centre asking for part-time help. There were ten replies so I've decided to interview the ones I think will be the most suitable.

I know I'll get muddled and forget what to ask if I don't have something to jog my memory when I see them. I've written down some questions on a sheet of paper in black biro leaving enough space between each question to give me room to write my comments and impressions on the interviewee's answers. I made several copies at the library when I went out.

Saturday, 25 May
The interviews went well. I looked at their CV, asked the questions and jotted down my comments. Afterwards I was able to reflect on the suitability of the applicants. Three of the candidates seemed to be just what I was looking for. I phoned all three and asked them to come and meet Faith. When I'd done that I phoned their last employers for references. After the candidates had met Faith, I engaged a girl called Blossom but both of the others agreed to help out in an emergency if they were free at the time.

Blossom was a Jamaican lady who had been a full-time care assistant in a local nursing home. She had left a year ago because she had broken her leg in an accident. She has now fully recovered.

She was pleased to be offered an interview for the post of temporary care assistant and presented herself, neat and tidy, at the appointed time. She found the interview straightforward and answered the questions truthfully. She was told the post was only temporary because of the nature of Faith's illness.

We discussed her hourly rate of pay, the hours she would work, meals

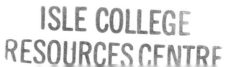

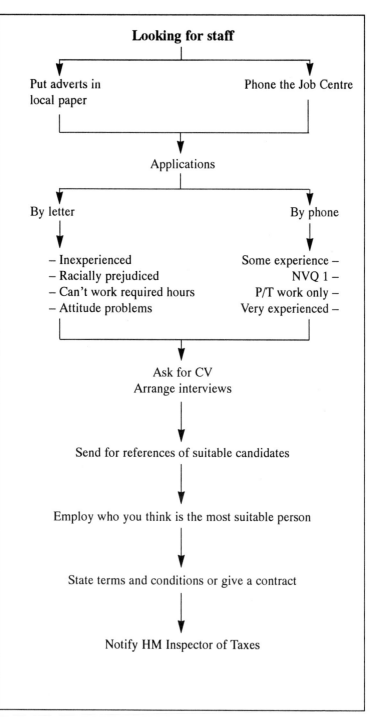

Fig. 15. Procedure for looking for staff.

Interview check sheet

Name of candidate   Date

Date of birth   Single/Married/Widow(er)/Divorced
How many children at home?
Hold old are they?

Applicant's address

CV seen – comments

Explain what the job entails before asking the questions

Why do you want a temporary job in a private house?

What experience have you had?

Are you in good health?

Do you have any other commitments?

What hours can you work?

Do you need any time off for booked holidays or appointments *etc*?

Are you willing to work at weekends and bank holidays?

Do you have any problems about caring for a terminally ill person?

Do you have any racial problems about caring for a Jamaican lady?

What hourly rate of pay are you hoping for?

If I employ you, when can you start?

How will you get here? Drive? Y/N Public transport? Y/N

Is there anything you would like to ask?

Comments:

Fig. 16. An interview sheet.

while she was on duty and what the work entailed. She would not be allowed any holiday until she was no longer needed but then she would be given an appropriate sum of money to cover all holidays that she had earned.

There was an instant rapport between Faith and Blossom and both looked forward to knowing each other more fully.

Keeping Grace's weight normal

The doctor had told Sally that people suffering from Parkinson's disease were not exempt from the other diseases that often plague elderly people. He had explained that while cancer and rheumatoid arthritis are not so common in people with Parkinson's disease, osteoarthritis could be a problem.

He had advised Grace not to put on any more weight. She should have a high fibre diet that includes plenty of fruit and vegetables. This kind of diet coupled with three or four glasses of water each day would also help to prevent the constipation that Grace was prone to.

The doctor advised against a high protein diet because this can affect the absorption of some of the drugs used for Parkinson's disease.

Grace liked all kinds of fruit and most vegetables but now found it difficult to bite into fruit. The housekeeper overcame this by making fruit salads or serving a single fruit cut up, topped with low fat yoghurt or fromage frais.

Scalding tea tips over Hannah's legs

Diary entry: Tuesday, 20 August
I was alone when I had the accident but fortunately I knew what to do. I'd just made myself a mug of lemon tea. I lifted it to my mouth and it slipped out of my fingers. The scalding liquid poured down my chest and tummy and over my legs. I couldn't feel my legs burning but I yelled with pain as the tea hit my chest. I wheeled myself into my new shower and turned on cold water and drenched myself through my clothes. Staying under the shower I called for help through my community alarm pendant which hung round my neck, fortunately it hadn't got wet. I was still in the shower when the ambulance came to take me to the accident and emergency department at our local hospital. Although they wrapped me in a blanket my wet clothing left a trail of water as I was taken out on a stretcher.

The siren was blaring and blue lights flashing. I would have enjoyed it if I hadn't been shivering with fear and cold, but the ambulance men were very kind and we soon arrived.

My husband was notified and came direct to the hospital but didn't arrive until after I had been admitted to the ward. He was a worried man but was assured that due to the cold shower it was unlikely that any lasting damage had been done. However, I will be kept in for a few days, just in case.

DISCUSSION POINTS

1. Who will be responsible for hiring and firing staff?

2. Who will be responsible for keeping the house clean?

3. Is it necessary to have a housekeeper or a gardener?

4. How many staff are needed to care for your sick relative?

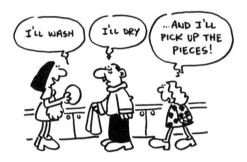

7
Looking at Finances

In this chapter the following will be discussed:

● calculating income

● allocating the money

● applying for benefits

● asking for a grant.

CALCULATING INCOME

Income may depend on:

● age (because some pensions increase with age)

● disabilities

● interest from invested capital (if any)

● interest from shares (if any)

● pensions, for example retirement, private, superannuation *etc*

● any salary received

● benefits from DSS

● rents from leased properties (including holiday accommodation).

Some of your relative's income may be paid on a weekly, monthly, quarterly or annual basis. When assessing income don't forget to include *all* monies paid to them throughout the year. See the calculation of income in Figure 17.

When you know what the income is you will have to decide which is the best way to use it – to find out if it will pay for everything or whether financial help will be needed either on a short-term or long-term basis.

Eric		£ p
Sate retirement pension		62.50
Attendance Allowance (AA)		32.40
	Total:	94.90
Alice (his sister)		
State pension:		33.50
Home work		20.00
	Total:	53.50

Eric's owns his house outright. This is not counted in his financial assessment. He has no capital. There is no charge for day care or other services from Social Services.

Fig. 17. Calculation of weekly income.

Faith's income

Anne applied for the care component of the Disability Living Allowance as soon as the doctor certified that she had less than six months to live. Because of her prognosis she did not have to fulfil any other conditions before it could be awarded.

Anne has also applied for income support for her sister and these are the allowances she thinks she will be given

		£ p
Disability Living Allowance (DLA)		48.50
Income Support		18.50
	Total:	67.00

She has £2,000 in the bank which she is prepared to use to pay for extra help if needed. There is no charge for the community nurse or the MacMillan nurses. Help from social services will probably be free of charge.

Grace's financial situation

Grace has no financial problems and pays for all her carers out of her own income which is around £1,000 per week.

	£ p
Approximate weekly income:	
Interest on capital	25.00
Rent from leased properties	800.00
State pension	65.00
Private pension	95.00
Dividends from shares	10.00
Total:	£995.00

She will be liable to pay income tax.

Hannah and Doug's weekly income

	£ p
Disability Living Allowance	48.50
Doug's salary	250.00 (after deductions)
	298.50

Doug is in the process of trying to claim for the invalid care allowance. Carers who spend more than 35 hours a week looking after someone who is disabled can apply for this allowance.

Please note: The above illustrations are fictitious examples. You must ask your relative's care manager to carry out a proper financial assessment and advise you of the outcome. The care manager will tell you what they can provide and how much, if anything, it will cost.

ALLOCATING THE MONEY

When you're deciding how to allocate the income you will find it similar to budgeting for your own household. You will probably find it easier to assess the cost of fixed outgoings, such as electricity, and put a weekly sum away for these bills.

Figure 18 is an example of outgoings which you may like to customise.

Services	Frequency of a/c	Approximate annual cost
Electricity	quarterly	x 4 = £
Gas	quarterly	x 4 = £
Telephone	quarterly	x 4 = £
Insurance	monthly	x 12 = £
Council tax	annual	£
Water rate	annual	£
Sewage rate	annual	£
Car licence	annual	£
Car insurance	annual	£
TV licence	annual	£
		÷ 52 =
		÷ 12 =

Add any other regular outgoings your relative has.

Fig. 18. List of regular outgoings.

Specific sums have not been put in as every household is different.

Suggestion: Put in your own approximate spending against each item. Add up the total and divide by twelve to get the monthly total or by 52 to get the weekly sum. Aim to put this sum of money away either weekly or monthly but remember that these totals will only be approximate. It's quite a good idea to put this money in a 'flex' or 'budget' account that pays interest on the balance but also allows the money to be used to pay the accounts.

Stamps can be used to pay specific service charges and these can be purchased from the post office if you prefer to pay by this method. For example you can buy stamps which can be used towards settling your gas or electricity account.

Buying food

Catering for one or two is often more expensive, per person, than providing meals for several people. Bear in mind that it generally costs more to buy small amounts. You may find it's more economical to buy larger quantities and freeze the surplus.

When freezing food take care that:

- correct procedures are followed for freezing food

- food is dated before freezing

- food is rotated by using the longest frozen first

- your appliances are kept clean

- your freezer is working properly and is freezing food to the correct temperature

- that the correct temperature for frozen food is maintained

- that you check frozen food regularly for signs of deterioration.

When buying food take into account your relative's:

- food preferences

- special diets

- food supplements such as 'Build Up' and 'Complan'

- food allergies

- difficulty with chewing or swallowing

- toleration of normal-size meals – he or she may need to have several small meals a day.

When buying food bear in mind also whether:

- you have appropriate storage facilities (fridge or freezer)

- time available for food preparation

- suitable cooking facilities.

Allowing for other expenses
When planning a budget make allowances for:

- hairdressing

- chiropody

- car fuel

- newspapers/magazines

- pet food

- clothing and footwear

- pharmacy items not covered by NHS prescriptions

- prescription charges if your relative is not exempt from paying.

The following are exempt from NHS prescription charges:

1. children up to the age of 16 or 18 if in full-time education

2. adults aged 60 and over

3. diabetics

4. those suffering from certain chronic diseases

5. expectant mothers

6. war pensioners.

You must sign the declaration on the back of NHS prescriptions verifying your relative is exempt from charges.

Applying to social services for services

Before help (services) can be given, a care needs assessment and a financial assessment must be carried out by a social worker – usually known as a care manager.

All doctor's surgeries have a special care manager to care for the needs of the elderly, the disabled, those with learning difficulties and other patients who have social problems. Many care managers visit the surgery, to which they are allocated, at regular intervals. They will meet carers and patients needing help or advice. Telephone the surgery to find out when they will be there. They can also be contacted at the local care manager's office.

The care manager will make an appointment to visit you and your relative to make the assessments. You, as the carer, can also have an assessment in your own right but you may have to ask for one. (Please refer to Chapter 10 – The Carers Act 1996, page 119).

The care manager will complete a care plan and will explain how much care your relative can expect to receive from social services. The financial side will also be explained and they will advise whether you should apply for income support for your relative.

APPLYING FOR BENEFITS

There are an abundance of booklets that will give explanations of the various benefits on offer. They can be obtained from the DSS offices, some post offices, Help the Aged and Age Concern. For all benefits there are forms to fill in. Precise information is required before an application can be considered. Forms can be obtained from your local Benefits Agency Offices. If you need guidance with filling them in make an appointment to talk to the manager at your local office. When you have completed the forms, post them in the envelope provided.

For some of the allowances your relative will be seen by an independent doctor who will make an assessment on behalf of the DSS.

Here are ten examples of questions the assessing doctor may ask:

1.   How good or bad is your relative's general health?

2.   What medicines and pills does your relative take?

3.   How mobile are they? – a demonstration may be asked for.

4.   Are they incontinent, of urine, faeces or both?

5.   How well do they sleep at night?

6.   How many times during the night and day do they need attention?

7.   How long have they been incapacitated?

8.   Do they have periods of confusion?

9.   How much can they do for themselves?

10. Can they get to the toilet and back unaided?

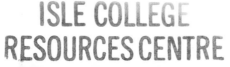

Answering the questions

Be prepared to answer to the best of your ability. This is sometimes difficult as sick people are often proud and tell the assessing doctor they are much more able than they really are. Some will deny they are incontinent because they feel ashamed.

Your records of your relative's activities, sleep pattern, how many times he or she needs attention during the night *etc* can be shown to the assessor.

Waiting for a reply

It may take several weeks following this assessment before you hear anything because all the information is discussed by a panel of professionals before a decision is made. In any case you have to be able to show that your relative has been incapacitated for six months before the benefit can be granted.

Ruling for the terminally ill

The six months rules does not apply if your relative has been diagnosed as having a terminal illness with a short life expectancy.

Keeping copies

Keep copies of all correspondence and reference numbers as letters and documents tend to get lost. Copies are useful to refer to if you are sent more forms to fill in. The average person finds it hard to remember exactly what they wrote down on the original form without something to refer to.

ASKING FOR A GRANT

There are many charities that are willing to help those in need. Most of them have certain criteria which must be fulfilled before the application can be considered.

Local charities often state that the applicant must live in a certain area – sometimes in a specific village! If you do not live there it's no use applying.

Others cater for applicants with certain illnesses such as multiple sclerosis. Some will help out with nursing home fees whilst others will give one-off grants for a specific purpose. They may for example, give something towards a computer that will help a person communicate. Some may help with clothing grants or pay something towards an outing. This kind of grant is usually geared towards children with severe or a terminal illness such as leukaemia.

Finding charities that offer help

To find out about the charities try the reference section of the main library in your area. If they haven't got a book of charities the librarian will try to order one for you from another library. It may take a few days to arrive and it will cost a small sum of money (about 50 pence). The Citizens' Advice Bureau usually know about local charities and may help you draft a letter of application.

Waiting

Special meetings are set aside to discuss the merits of each application. You will be notified if they are able to offer your relative any financial assistance. It may take some time before you get their decision.

CASE STUDIES

Assessing Eric's finances

Diary entry: Tuesday, 21 May
Miss Smith the care manager also did a financial assessment during her visit today.

First of all she asked about his income: his state pension, allowances and benefits. Then she wanted to know about his outgoings: how much mortgage or rent he paid *etc*.

I thought she would ask a lot of questions so I found out all about his financial state (there wasn't much to find out) and wrote it all down. It made things easier. I did get caught out on his post office savings book though. I didn't know he had one. I was pleased to discover he had £50 in the account.

The care manager said that although he owns his house it would not affect the assessment as it didn't count as capital. His savings, which amount to £2,000 approximately, were too low to be taken into account. She told us that because Eric's income and savings were so low he wouldn't have to pay for the services they were providing.

Developing bedsores on Faith's sacrum

Diary entry: Saturday, 15 June
This morning we noticed that Faith's back looked red and sore despite all our constant care to her pressure areas. This is very disheartening. Our MacMillan nurse says that it's probably due to lack of proper food – she's not eating at all now.

Faith doesn't seem to feel any discomfort but that's probably because the strength of the drugs had to be increased yesterday to control her other pain. All we can do is to keep turning her and treating her pressure areas to try and prevent more sores developing.

We did get her a spenco mattress a few weeks ago, I'm sure that has helped. After she was incontinent last week, nurse inserted a catheter into her bladder so she would be spared incontinence and the effort of getting onto a bedpan. I hate seeing Faith like this but my feelings are mixed. I want to keep her and care for her but I also want her to die for her own sake. She told me one day that she's not afraid as she will be with her Lord. I don't know quite what she meant – I must ask her pastor when he comes.

Faith seems to have lapsed into unconsciousness now and isn't aware of anything or anybody. Her friends from the church came again – they come every day and just sit there holding her hand to read to her and pray.

It can't be long now.

Sunday, 16 June, evening
The pastor called after morning service and sat with Faith for a short while. He asked if I was alright before he left and said he would be back tomorrow unless I wanted him to come sooner. The doctor and the MacMillan nurse called. They were very kind and will come if I need them. It was a busy morning but the afternoon was quiet. I just sat with Faith and held her hand. She knew I was there.

She opened her eyes just once and said, 'Thank you Anne'. It broke my heart.

As I watched, her eyes closed again and her face took on a look of joy. She didn't wake again. She has gone to be with her Lord.

Grace becomes constipated

Grace was feeling bloated and uncomfortable. She had not opened her bowels for several days. Her senior carer had increased the amount of fluids she already drank and had given her bran with her breakfast cereal but it seemed that this wasn't enough. She decided to inform the doctor and ask his advice.

The doctor explained that constipation was a symptom of Parkinson's disease and was caused by the movement of her bowel muscles slowing down. The condition was made worse because Grace was not as physically active as somebody who doesn't suffer from Parkinson's disease. He looked at Grace's drugs and said that the medicines she was taking might be making her constipation worse. However, as they were giving Grace a reasonable quality of life he would continue to prescribe them for her.

He also prescribed dioctyl solution to be taken twice a day and some fybogel sachets. The contents to be mixed in half a glass of water, or fruit juice. (Fybogel must be drunk as soon as it is mixed otherwise it will quickly set into a gel.) This was to be taken once a day to start with but could be increased up to three times daily if necessary. 'Drinking water comes out of the tap and Grace should be encouraged to drink more,' the doctor said. He also suggested that the carer should see the dietician to discuss whether Grace's diet could be improved.

The carer was told that laxatives shouldn't be given if Grace passed three or more motions a week as excessive use of laxatives could lead to other complications. But if constipation wasn't treated it would become so severe that it might lead to difficulty in passing urine, incontinence and confusion, particularly at night.

The doctor asked to be informed if her condition improved. Otherwise she may need suppositories or an enema.

Within a few days she was feeling better. Her bowels had worked and her bloated feeling had gone.

Hannah needs treatment

Hannah's periods were less frequent now but when she did have one it was heavy, prolonged and left her feeling drained and exhausted. Coupled with this problem she had started to have hot flushes which were not only uncomfortable but embarrassing if she was in company. She phoned the surgery and asked for a visit from her lady doctor. The doctor was sympathetic. She prescribed some tablets to help control the menopausal symptoms and also referred Hannah to a gynaecologist for investigation of her problems.

DISCUSSION POINTS

1. Will your relative's income supply all his or her care needs?

2. Should the family apply to social services for help?

3. Should the family consider applying for a grant?

4. Can any members of the family help to support their sick relative financially?

8
Caring for the Terminally Ill

In this chapter the following will be discussed:

- giving information

- feelings of the family

- attending to final details

- arranging the funeral

- disposal of belongings.

GIVING INFORMATION

Before your relative can be told about their prognosis there are a number of considerations.

- Whether they want to know how long they are going to live.

- Who should tell them about their expectation of life?

- Do you have accurate knowledge of the situation?

- Should the doctor or nurse be involved?

- Whether you, your relative or the rest of the family need the care of hospice nurses.

Many people feel that if someone has only a short time to live, they have a right to know. It is certainly right to tell the person concerned if he or she wants to know.

They may want to make their peace with God or use the time they have left to see all their family and friends for one last time. Some want to say sorry for a hurt they caused in the past, while others may have 'things' they would like to finish.

But what about those who don't want to hear about their impending death? If you tell this kind of person you might:

● take away their reason for living

● make all their aches and pains seem to get worse

● cause them to give up

● make them feel depressed.

Deciding who's going to tell

Assuming that it has been decided to give this kind of information to your relative it then has to be discussed who will tell them. It could be:

● the doctor

● nurse or MacMillan nurse (hospice movement)

● a member of the family or a valued friend

● yourself as the carer – this is generally unlikely unless you are a relative.

Then it has to be decided when and how the information should be given. There is no right time, right person or right way in which your relative should be told. Everybody has their own ideas. Each person is an individual. The way of telling must be tailored to be the least painful way for both your relative and the person giving the information. Many sick people realise that they will not recover but keep it to themselves to spare their loved ones. Some know but refuse to accept the situation, whilst others have no idea about the state of their health.

Considering your relative's feelings
It really depends on your relative's attitude how they react to the news of their impending death. Some will accept it and carry on doing the things they want to do as far as they are able.

Others will be shocked and disbelieving. They may start to grieve for the life they are losing. Some will put it to the back of their mind – they don't want to know about such things! Most people are generally saddened because they will not be able to see their children or grand-children develop. They think of lost opportunities that will never return, wrongs they have done that they may not have time to make right and other things they are desperate to do but now have no time.

Your relative's doctor should be informed of the intention to tell your relative. There could be adverse affects, for example depressive illness that will need his help and care.

Changing needs

Although many people think of a terminally ill patient as being a person who is very sick and bed-bound this is not necessarily so. Many people with terminal cancer are active and appear to be 'healthy' until the last few days. Some patients' health declines slowly, others deteriorate rapidly.

The needs of a relative suffering from terminal illness will change as their health fails. At first they may be independent, washing and dressing themselves, walking about and doing most things that a well person might do. At this time they may need little more help than the reassurance and company you provide.

They may be given palliative treatment to alleviate symptoms, such as the pain caused by cancer, but it will not cure the problem.

As the disease progresses your relative will become more dependent on you and look to you, as their carer, for both physical and psycholog-ical help and comfort.

Being referred to a hospice

If your relative is suffering from terminal cancer or AIDS the doctor can refer him or her to the MacMillan or hospice nurses. They are experts in caring for terminally ill patients both in the hospice and in the commu-nity. If he omits to do this *ask* for a referral to be made. The advantages of this are:

- Your relative will be assessed as a whole person.

- Physical and mental pain will be assessed.

- Recommended pain control will be discussed with the doctor.

- There will be on-going assessment of symptoms and pain control.

- Medications will be constantly reviewed.

- Bereavement counselling will be available to the patient, their family and carers.

- The hospice/MacMillan nurses make regular and emergency calls.

- They can, if necessary, recommend admission to the hospice to control intractable pain and other symptoms.

- Hospice/MacMillan nurses also work closely with the patient, family, doctor and carer.

- They help all people concerned but never intrude.

- If necessary they will continue to help the family after death.

- This service is available under the NHS.

CONSIDERING THE FEELINGS OF THE FAMILY

Parents are usually the centre of most families until the children start their own families. After this the parents move from the centre but remain very close as they are loved by grandchildren as well. The feelings of the close-knit family nucleus will be shock and sadness.

Close relatives or friends feel that they want to protect their loved ones from any kind of hurt, almost to the point where they smother them. Others start to grieve as soon as they hear the news and fail to hide their distress. This can cause their sick relative to feel guilty because they are going to die. (This could happen to your relative.)

Worrying

Spouses worry about the future:

- How will they manage without their other half?

- How will they cope with the loneliness?

- Will they cope with shopping and keeping the house clean?

They will also feel stunned, shocked and angry, asking 'Why me?'.

Unmarried partners, particularly homosexual partners, may have their own particular worries:

- Will they be accepted as part of the family when it comes to making funeral arrangements?

- Will they be blamed for a loved son's terminal illness caused by AIDS?

- Will they be allowed to continue caring during their sick partner's final weeks?

The stigma of homosexuality still exists and some people find it difficult to hide their feelings at a time of pending loss.

ATTENDING TO FINAL DETAILS

When your relative passes away you will need to notify the doctor as soon as possible after the death. However, few doctors appreciate being called out to certify a death when it happens during the night. It might be wiser to call him or her before surgery the following morning. You could ask your relative's doctor which he or she would prefer beforehand.

Referring a death to the coroner

Providing the doctor does not have to refer the death to the coroner he or she will give you a certificate stating the cause of your relative's death. This is to be taken to the registrar when you register the death. Referral to the coroner is likely to happen if a person dies:

- in suspicious circumstances

- within one year of having an operation

- unexpectedly

- by committing suicide

- within a year following a serious accident.

The doctor will ask if your relative's body is for burial or cremation. The body of the deceased must be examined by another doctor and a special form signed before cremation can take place.

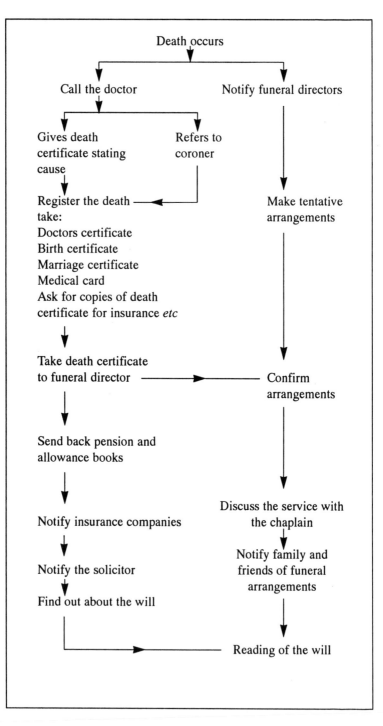

Fig. 19. Procedure following a death.

Notifying the funeral director

While you are waiting for the doctor to arrive contact your chosen funeral director. He will take the deceased to the chapel of rest as soon as death has been certified.

You will be asked:

● the full name (and maiden name if applicable) of the deceased

● your relative's date of birth

● date and time of death

● where the body is at the present time

● whether the deceased is for burial, cremation or other form of disposal.

You will also have to give the undertaker a death certificate given to you by the registrar. Then arrangements can be finalised.

Figure 19 acts as a summary of the procedure following a death.

ARRANGING THE FUNERAL

Discuss with the funeral director:

● the wishes of the deceased

● date, time and place of the funeral

● special form of service (choice of hymns, prayers, readings *etc*)

● religious requirements of their faith (Roman Catholic; Jewish; Muslim *etc*)

● the chaplain whom you would like to take the service

● the church at which the service is to be held (if any)

● transport for the immediate family

● prearranged funeral arrangements (if applicable)

● fees and costs

● any other queries you may have.

Note: Discuss the form of service with whoever is chosen to conduct the service.

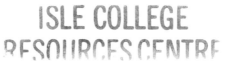

Notifying others
Remember that you may need to notify the following:

1. *DSS – pensions* if your relative received a pension

2. *DSS – allowances* if your relative received any allowances

3. DSS to apply for *state benefits*

4. *private pension funds* – if applicable

5. the appropriate *life policy insurance company*

6. any *credit companies* that money is owed to

7. any *hire-purchase company* money is owed to

8. *credit card companies* that your relative has been using

9. your relative's *solicitor* (if they have one)

10. *HM Inspector of Taxes* if appropriate

11. your relative's *care manager*

12. *banks, Giro or building societies* where accounts are held

13. *car licensing authorities* (if they had a driving licence).

Sending out invitations
Most families make arrangements for the funeral guests to receive refreshments before returning to their homes. The simplicity or lavishness of the occasion depends on:

● the wishes of the deceased

● family feelings

- finances

- available premises.

The family will decide where the venue shall be. This might be at the home of the deceased, the home of a relative, a hall or hotel. They will also decide on the menu and who will serve it and clear away afterwards.

Send RSVP invitations to relatives and friends who you wish to invite to have refreshments afterwards. Others can be invited to the service and ceremony only.

Wording the invitations

When planning the invitation make sure you include the following details on the card:

- name of the deceased

- date, time and place of funeral

- time and place of crematorium (if applicable)

- place where to gather afterwards

- special instructions regarding flowers or donations to a charity

- your name and address for RSVP.

It's useful to send a map to mourners living outside the area.

Reading the will

Years ago the will used to be read at the house immediately after the funeral. Nowadays, if a solicitor is dealing with this matter it is usually read at his office.

It can, however, be read at any time or place that is convenient to the beneficiaries. If an executor has already been appointed that person will be responsible for sorting out details of bequests. He or she should also ensure that each beneficiary gets their entitlement and be responsible for the distribution of any mementoes.

If no one has been appointed it is up to the family to select somebody who is willing and capable of doing the job.

Probate

If there is no will it would be wise to consult a solicitor regarding current law on probate.

DISTRIBUTING THE BELONGINGS

The deceased's last will and testament has to be read before anything can be disposed of.

Once all the clauses of the will have been satisfied everything else can be sorted and distributed to beneficiaries, given away or sold. If there is no valid will nothing can be disposed of until written permission is granted from the probate office or your solicitor.

It's always upsetting to have to dispose of a loved one's home when they have passed away. Try to share this onerous task with another member of the family or a friend who will support you.

Consulting a solicitor

Consult a solicitor if:

● no valid will is found

● when property or other valuable items need to be sold

● if no executor has been appointed

● if any other legal problems arise.

Selling vehicles

You can sell a car privately but it must be in good condition and should have a current MOT Certificate if it's over three years old. Some buyers return again and again if they find the slightest fault. If the vehicle is not roadworthy you can approach a garage to dispose of it or a breakers yard where it can be broken up for spare parts. Some vintage cars are valuable. Take advice before selling. Remember to notify the vehicle registration office when the car has been disposed of.

Giving away the furniture

Try:

● asking family and friends if they would like any pieces

- charitable organisations such as the Salvation Army of WRVS

- approaching local charity shops.

Selling the furniture
Try:

- advertising the items in the local paper

- auction rooms – an estate agent many be able to advise

- a garage sale

- local car boot sales, if you have transport

- second-hand shops that do house clearance.

  Remember it is illegal to sell faulty electrical items.

Disposal of clothing

1. Nearly new shops will take good clothing to sell giving you a percentage of the price received.

2. Charity shops take all manner of goods to sell for the charity they represent and may be able to arrange collection of the goods.

3. Crises in any part of the world call for donations of clothing with details regarding collection. Clothing needs to be suitable for the purpose for which it is required. For example, there's no point in sending posh evening wear to a community that has just suffered an earthquake or severe flooding.

4. Seasonal appeals, for example Crisis at Christmas. London and some of the large towns have temporary seasonal centres for the homeless. Here, they are given food, bathing facilities and good clean clothing before they leave.

5. Local groups that hold jumble sales to raise funds. Try the local Scout Troop.

CASE STUDIES

Alice looks into prearranged funeral arrangements

Diary entry: Monday, 27 May
It occurred to me over the weekend that Eric and I are the last living members of our family. It set me thinking about our funerals. I know that we both decided years ago to be cremated, but who will be there to make arrangements? Neither of us have any close friends so what should we do?

I have seen several advertisements for prearranged funerals so I thought I would find out more about them.

Today I phoned the local undertaker who said he had a scheme of his own and would send me details. He also offered to come round and explain everything once I'd seen his brochure.

Later I went to the post office to collect our pensions and found a leaflet in there. Looking through some magazines I discovered adverts for other schemes. I've sent off for all the information and will try and decide which is the best scheme for us.

The main advantages seem to be:

1. We will pay less if we prearrange our funerals.

2. We can choose what we want beforehand.

3. We know our wishes will be carried out as fast as possible.

4. We don't have to leave money (which might not be enough) to pay for something that will happen when we're dead.

5. Our funerals won't be a burden on the state or anybody else.

6. We can either pay the complete cost now or pay by instalments.

I've been worrying about what will happen to our bodies. Once I've chosen the right scheme and paid for this service I shall feel easier in my mind about it.

Anne registers Faith's death

Diary entry: Monday, 17 June
Once the doctor had certified Faith's death he asked whether she was to be buried or cremated. Apparently, another certificate has to be com-

pleted and signed by himself and another doctor before cremation. I told him that Faith had always preferred the thought of being cremated. I had already contacted the funeral director; he came just after the doctor had left. Our doctor said his colleague would see Faith at the funeral parlour later today.

Before he left the doctor gave me a certificate stating the cause of her death which I would need to take to the registrar.

Once the office of registration was open I took the doctor's certificate, Faith's medical card, birth and marriage certificate to the registrar. I didn't need an appointment but I might have needed one in a different district.

The registrar was very kind, offering her condolences and a tissue when I broke down and cried. She gave me another certificate which I took to the undertaker. The funeral has now been booked for next Friday at twelve noon. When I got home I notified the pastor of her church who agreed to officiate at the service.

I managed to get most of the invitations out today. I don't quite know what to do about her husband because up until now he hasn't known my address. To be quite honest, I'm a bit afraid of him! I suppose I could invite him to the church service and crematorium only.

Grace has a 'flu jab

Diary entry: Thursday, 3 October
When I went to pick up a prescription for Grace at the surgery I noticed they were making arrangements to give 'flu vaccinations for the coming winter. When I enquired about Grace the receptionist put her name down and told me the doctor would visit and give it to her at home. When he called, he asked if Grace was feeling well and examined her throat and lungs before he gave the injection. There was no reaction to the vaccine and it should protect her against having any nasty doses of 'flu this winter.

Hannah donates her body to medical science

Diary entry: Monday, 26 August
I've often thought I would like to do something useful with my body after I die. So the other day I phoned HM Inspector of Anatomies' office for details. They told me that many people donate their bodies for medical science but when the time comes some are not accepted. However, he agreed to send me the necessary forms.

The documents arrived today so I discussed the matter with Doug this evening. He didn't like the idea as arrangements would be made to transfer my body to the appropriate centre immediately my death has been certified. He felt that the family should be responsible for my funeral arrangements rather than the anatomy office. They will dispose of my body as they feel is most appropriate. There won't be a charge for this service.

I told him that he could still arrange my funeral after they had finished the research if he wanted to but he would have to bear the cost. Doug felt happier about that and told me that if that was what I wanted, to go ahead.

We filled in the forms and returned them. We've told everybody who is involved in my care what procedure to take in the event of my death.

DISCUSSION POINTS

● How much do you feel your dying relative should be told about their prognosis?

● Are you aware of your relative's wishes regarding his or her funeral *etc*?

● Do you know whether they have made a will?

● Do you know where the will has been lodged?

9
Picking Up the Pieces

In this chapter the following will be discussed:

● grieving

● counselling

● getting help from organisations

● starting again

● helping other people.

GRIEVING

Having time to think

The funeral is over, the guests have gone. The will has been read and your much loved relative's belongings have been sorted and disposed of. During this time you have probably been busy, seeing people, making sure that everything gets to the right person, particularly if you are the executor.

Now it's over, you have time to sit and think.

Seeing fewer friends

Unless you have a job and go out to work you may find that you see few other people at this time. You wonder why they never come near you now it's all over. You think they feel embarrassed because they don't know how to handle bereavement. If they meet you in the street they may greet you with downcast eyes, give a quick greeting and maybe ask how you are. They will expect you say, that you're fine. You oblige them and tell them you're alright. You present a 'stiff upper lip' because you don't want anybody to know how bad you really feel.

How are you feeling?

You may be experiencing isolation and loneliness with only your thoughts to turn to.

Suddenly, you feel exhausted. It's too much trouble to get up and get a decent meal together; anyway you're not feeling hungry.

You may not be sleeping properly but you tell yourself it's because you haven't had much to do since Mum, Dad or Auntie died. You probably don't feel you need to go to your doctor because you're not really ill. Days and weeks pass, you're not sleeping any better, the exhaustion is still there.

Feeling irritable and angry

You snap if anybody offers you advice and then chide yourself afterwards. The snappiness turns to anger against everything and everybody. Even God gets His fair share: 'Why did it happen to me? Why take my Mum? She didn't do anybody any harm, I loved her God. Why didn't you take someone that nobody loves?'

Feeling guilty

You find yourself crying, it's difficult to stop. You're overwhelmed with feelings of guilt: 'If only I'd done more to help Mum. If I hadn't gone on holiday, Mum would be here now. I should have noticed she was ill,' and so on.

Widows may feel they pushed their husbands too far; nagging him to mow the lawn when he should have been resting. Nagging him to finish the decorating quickly or something similar.

Grieving later

Some people do not appear to grieve at all – at least not until much later.

Delayed grieving can come when everybody thinks you have come to terms with your loss. Fortunately this doesn't happen very often, but if it does occur the grieving can be prolonged and may be more difficult to overcome.

COUNSELLING

It's important to recognise what you are going through is part of the pattern of grieving. You may need help to enable you to come to terms with your grief and loss.

Go and talk to your doctor. He will almost certainly suggest that you see a bereavement counsellor. Don't be afraid, it doesn't mean that you're insane. It offers a way to recovery – of coming to terms with your loss so you can carry on with your life. Some surgeries offer a counselling service but others haven't got this facility. In this case you will be referred to the nearest counselling service.

Counselling usually takes several sessions. Recovery can't be hurried but you will feel progressively better and more able to cope.

GETTING HELP FROM ORGANISATIONS

The Samaritans
The Samaritans are at the end of a telephone 24 hours a day, seven days a week including bank holidays. Your local branch telephone number will be in the telephone directory. It doesn't matter what time it is when you feel the need of a sympathetic listener, you will find one by phoning the Samaritans.

Every person who works for this voluntary organisation has been specially trained to help you, without giving unwanted advice.

You will be asked for your name but you do not have to give your proper name. Choose one that the Samaritan you speak to can call you by because it's difficult to have a discussion with a nameless person! Conversations are always confidential. However, if you are contemplating immediate suicide you will be asked if somebody can come and be with you.

Samaritans' offices are open during the day and welcome clients who want to drop in and talk about their problems with one of the volunteers.

CRUSE
Cruse is an organisation which trains their members to help a bereaved person to come to terms with their new status. In some cases this will involve helping a person who has had to go through a change of role.

Example
When a young mother dies the father may have to take over as mother and father to his children. He may even have to give up his job and income to look after them.

MacMillan and Hospice at Home nurses
MacMillan and Hospice at Home nurses are trained to give counselling to their bereaved families and carers. They usually do follow-up visits after the death has occurred. They may advise you to see a counsellor for help on a regular basis until you feel able to cope again.

Other counselling services
There may be other organisations in your area that offer a counselling service. Some churches have set up bereavement counselling groups run by trained people: Ask at the:

● doctor's surgery

● town information centre

● local churches

● Citizens' Advice Bureau

● library.

Warning: It is not advisable to go to unqualified people who advertise themselves as counsellors.

STARTING AGAIN

The first steps towards making a new start are always the worst. Once you begin to do some of the things you did before you will begin to feel better.

Joining an exercise class is one way to improve your health, make new friends and help you feel more cheerful. Exercise is said to release hormones in your body that gives you a feeling of wellbeing. Gentle exercise is best at the beginning – you can always graduate to the more strenuous stuff later. You should check with your doctor that you are physically fit enough to join any fitness class.

Take up your old hobbies or try your hand at new ones. Hobbies give you interest; group hobbies introduce you to new friends.

Going back to business
Returning to work often helps, but you may find that you need a new, more challenging job. It's never easy to find or change employment but look round for something suitable and apply. Don't be discouraged if you don't succeed at first, keep on trying – think of it as a new challenge.

HELPING OTHER PEOPLE

Bereavement is an awful experience to go through but the experience of coming to terms with loss and grief yourself can be used to help others. You may be interested in applying to join one of the counselling organisations such as CRUSE. You will, of course, be interviewed but will not be eligible to join as a trainee counsellor immediately. Two years must pass following your bereavement before you can be accepted for training.

The Samaritans welcome helpers who can give a few hours a week but volunteers have to attend an initial training course (by the Samaritans). This teaches them how best to answer the phones and talk to clients who are seeking help.

After being interviewed, trained and accepted a period of working under supervision always follows. Nobody is ever left to cope on their own.

CASE STUDIES

Alice, Eric's sister, has to go in hospital

Diary entry: Tuesday, 4 June
I woke up this morning feeling ill. My tongue was dry and furry and I had such a pain in my tummy. I thought I would feel better if I went to the toilet. Even when I'd washed and cleaned my teeth I felt awful and went back to bed for a bit. I dozed off to sleep again and woke to hear Eric calling me. I went to him but thankfully, at that moment Eric's carer arrived to get him ready to go to day care. Jenny, his carer for the day, saw me and told me I looked awful. Before I knew it, she had taken me back to bed and called the doctor. By the time he arrived the pain had moved to my right side and I felt worse than ever.

Jenny phoned the social services and asked permission to stay with me after Eric had gone.

The doctor said I had appendicitis and had to have my appendix out. As he phoned the ambulance service he assured me I would only be in hospital a few days. What will happen to Eric?

Jenny phoned social services and informed them what had happened. They asked Jenny to pack some clothes for Eric as they would admit him to a residential home for a few weeks until I was well enough to care for him again.

Jenny also packed a case for me and promised she would come and visit while I was in hospital.

Anne goes through the grieving process

Diary entry: Friday, 28 June
The funeral is over, Faith's belongings have been disposed of. Much to my surprise Faith's husband hasn't caused any problems, in fact he seemed quite stricken with grief and guilt.

The house is too quiet. I keep going into Anne's room thinking she's still there and then bursting into tears when she isn't. Then I grow angry:

why has God taken my only sister who was so gentle and kind? Why my sister? But of course I don't know the answer.

Then I feel guilty. I should have known that she was ill and that she was in pain. Why hadn't I noticed that she used to drench herself in perfume? It wasn't like her.

Friday, 12 July

I must buck myself up. I don't feel that I want to go anywhere or do anything. The house is in a state and the weeds are growing so fast they've almost taken over.

Our MacMillan nurse called in this morning to see if I was alright. It was sweet of her. We had a cup of tea and we talked about Faith and the funeral, I showed her the photos I'd taken. She suggested that I contacted CRUSE. She'd given me the number. Apparently CRUSE is an organisation that helps bereaved people to come to terms with their loss.

Wednesday, 16 October

I'm feeling better about Faith's death now. CRUSE have helped me a lot. I still have my special person that I can phone if I get a bad episode but those are getting less and less now.

The pastor of Faith's church has visited and invited me to go there on Sunday. He's even arranged for somebody to fetch me. I'm not a churchgoer but I think I shall go this Sunday.

Grace has a nose bleed

Milly, Grace's carer, had just given Grace her 'elevenses' and gone into the kitchen to get herself a cup of coffee. Coming back into the lounge she saw her wiping her hand across her face and blood everywhere. Grace was bleeding from her nose.

Milly reassured her and called to the housekeeper to bring a bowl of water, some towels and cloths. She held the soft part of Grace's nose – where it joins the bony part telling her to breathe through her mouth. When the housekeeper brought the bowl of water she tried to get Grace to bend over it to catch any dripping blood. This was difficult because her back muscles were rather rigid. For the next ten minutes the women supported Grace while Milly continued to apply gentle pressure to Grace's nose and to observe her condition.

Finally the bleeding stopped and Milly was able to wash Grace, change her dress and make her more comfortable.

Normally Milly would have protected her patient's clothing but in the few minutes she was out of the lounge Grace's clothing became quite bloodstained. There were no further episodes of bleeding but Milly knew that if it had started again Grace may have had to go to hospital for treatment.

She was careful not to give her any hot drinks for a few hours as this might have started the bleeding again.

Milly notified the doctor who said he would visit later that day.

Hannah has a friend to visit

Diary entry: Monday, 23 September
Because my friend, Julia, had been on holiday for a month it had been some time since I had seen her. It was about 2.30pm when she arrived. She said the journey had been tedious and stressful because there was so much traffic on the road.

Julia seemed to be acting out of character today, walking unsteadily, almost as though she'd had too much to drink and was drunk. I knew though, that she was teetotal!

When she sat down she didn't say much and didn't want to do anything, in fact she became quite lethargic.

I was puzzled until I remembered that Julia had told me once that she was a diabetic and had to have insulin injections twice a day. Fortunately, Maureen, one of my carer's, was with me. As soon as I mentioned that Julia was diabetic she realised what was happening. She quickly fetched us both a fruit drink and helped Julia hold hers while she drank it. She told me later that she had put some extra sugar in it. Afterwards she gave us a sweet to suck while she went to get our afternoon tea.

Julia quickly recovered and thanked Maureen for her prompt action. She told us that because she wanted to get to us early she hadn't had any lunch and thought her blood sugar must have dropped too low.

We made sure that she had a proper meal and persuaded her to stay the night.

DISCUSSION POINTS

1. Do you feel that any of the mourners need counselling?

2. Have the feelings and grieving of the children been taken into account? Do you feel they would benefit from counselling to help them come to terms with their loss?

3. How do you feel you have coped with your grief? Do you think you could use your experience to help others through their grieving process?

10
Caring for the Carers

In this chapter the following will be discussed:

● assessing the needs of carers

● training carers

● supporting carers

● the Carer's Act 1996.

ASSESSING THE NEEDS OF CARERS

Looking at what carers would like

Most carers would like hospital conditions and equipment available wherever they work, whether in a private house or any other establishment. Indeed, if the carer has learnt his or her skills in a hospital they may find it difficult to adapt to a home situation.

Comparing home and hospital facilities

Some prescribed treatment needs equipment available in a hospital ward, for example a drip, suction or dialysis machine. In the ordinary household it is more difficult to get the necessary apparatus. It may have to be hired, borrowed or purchased and can take weeks to arrive. In the meantime the carer has to improvise.

Again in hospital, carers can always call on another person to help carry out a task whereas at home they have to work alone most of the time.

If a carer works in hospital he or she can be almost sure of getting off duty on time. However, working in a private house means having to wait for somebody to come and relieve him or her. If this doesn't happen for any reason the carer is unable to leave until a replacement is found. Carers, like everybody else, want to be able to arrange their leisure time knowing that, unless there is a real emergency, they can get off duty on time.

Wearing protective clothing

If you work in a hospital or nursing home you are given a uniform, plastic aprons and gloves to protect you and your clothing from infection and spills.

Agency staff are also required to wear uniform whilst on duty but private carers often use their normal clothing. However, sometimes protective clothing is necessary. Chemists sell or will get disposable aprons and gloves to order. Either buy them yourself or if you're employed ask your employers to buy aprons and gloves for you. Use them for work that might cause soiling or pollution, for example:

● giving and emptying bedpans or commodes

● bathing or washing the patient

● washing your relative's hair

● changing dressings

● emptying or changing urine and colostomy bags.

Considering the carer's personal needs

If a carer is employed by the family their needs, as an employee, will have been discussed when they were employed (see Chapter 3, page 38).

However, the carers who are friends or members of the family have no agreement or contract. They work long hours caring for their relative as well as doing all the other household jobs.

It is essential that other members of the family consider the basic needs of the carer who often gives love, care and hard work for no financial reward.

Most of us need:

● time for rest and leisure

● a room of our own

● a certain amount of privacy

● pocket money

● consideration and courtesy.

Carers are no different in this respect – they are individuals and have lives of their own. They may also have other commitments and additional personal needs, for example children to attend to. Others may also have to work for a salary as well as caring for a relative.

Considering the needs of the carer as well as the patient helps to promote harmony in the home.

GAINING EXPERIENCE AS A CARER

If extra help is required it is easier for your relative and the family to employ an experienced carer who knows what the job entails and how to do it because:

● Your relative will feel more confident and relaxed.

● The family will know their relative is being properly looked after.

● Family members will be able to learn from an experienced carer.

Many people who have the job of caring thrust upon them have no idea what taking total care of a sick person entails. They may like to consider getting some experience to help them in their new situation.

You may feel that either you don't need to gain experience or that you haven't the time to learn – but it's worth the effort. The advantages of gaining some experience will:

● help you cope with accidents such as falls and abrasions

● show you how to lift patients without straining your back

● teach you useful techniques

● help you deal with emotional outbursts and difficult people

● help you to devise workable routines

● show you how to work with other people

● teach you how to demonstrate techniques to carers less able than yourself.

There are a number of ways of gaining experience.

1. Organisations such as the Red Cross and St John Ambulance Association run home nursing courses. Ask at your local branch for details. The courses are divided into sessions and run over several weeks.

2. Nursing homes sometimes employ inexperienced carers and they will be taught basic care by experienced staff. They often employ part-time as well as full-time staff. If you do not want permanent work in the home the matron may allow you to work on a voluntary basis for a few days.

3. Hospitals usually employ experienced carers but may allow you to work on a voluntary basis depending on hospital policy.

TRAINING FOR CARERS

Many establishments, including agencies, now require their carers to have obtained either their National Vocational Qualification (NVQ) or to be working towards it. Theory is taught and projects are set by the college tutors but practical work is learnt and assessed in the workplace.

There are varying grades of the NVQ, starting with Level One for absolute beginners. These and other similar courses are run at many education centres around the country.

Training therefore, can either be **informal** in order to gain experience or **formal**, leading to a recognised qualification (see Figure 20).

Informal	NVQ Levels 1–5	Nursing courses
No recognised certificates	Recognised certificate for each level	RGN certificate
Nursing home, residential home or hospital, may be as a volunteer	Education centre, hospital or nursing home for practical experience	

Fig. 20. Training for carers.

Learning can be costly
Carer's can undertake these courses free of charge (at present) provided they complete all the courses they undertake before they are twenty-five. Unfortunately, carers over this age, have to pay the full costs. Fees can be expensive. Make enquiries regarding cost and the commitment you will be expected to make before embarking on your NVQs.

SUPPORTING CARERS

Caring can be a very lonely and isolated job particularly if you are working alone. You need the support of friends and the rest of the family if you are caring for a relative. Carers working in hospitals or other caring establishments should receive support from their colleagues and senior staff.

Helping agencies to help their carers
Professional carers often work through nursing agencies. If there is a problem they are able to phone the agency and obtain help and advice. Agencies can register with the United Kingdom Home Care Association who aim to advise how to support and care for the carers they employ.

Working alone
The Carers National Association has been instrumental in bringing about the Carer's Act 1996. The Association is there for carers needing help, advice or information.

Apart from national organisations many local groups have been set up, for example 'Care for the Carers' covering Sussex.

Emergency alert card service
Organisations are there to support carers who care for sick or disabled relatives or friends. Some groups are able to offer carers an emergency alert service. The carer is given a card which they must carry with them whenever they leave the person they're caring for on his or her own. Should the carer be involved in an accident it ensures that the person being cared for will get help.

Get in touch with your local group and ask what support they offer. Such organisations produce informative leaflets, periodic magazines and some produce books on various aspects of caring.

To find out how to contact your local support group try:

● looking in the telephone directory

● asking at the library

- asking a nursing agency

- contacting the Citizens' Advice Bureau

- phoning the local council

- asking the community nurses

- looking on your doctor's surgery notice board

- asking other carers.

THE CARER'S (RECOGNITION AND SERVICES) ACT 1996

The original draft of the Carer's Bill entitled carers to obtain services for themselves. However, in order that the Bill could become an Act of Law that particular clause had to be omitted. The only service that a carer is entitled to a present, is that of having their own assessment. The assessment can only be given when the person you are caring for is being given a community care assessment by a social worker (care manager).

Carer assessments are not always automatically offered and you may have to ask for one. They are to determine what a carer needs to enable him or her to give a relative or friend the care needed to live as normal a life as possible.

Assessing you, the carer

The assessment will highlight any inadequacy in the care that you are able to give. The care manager will take into account:

- your **commitments** (for example, if you have children to care for)

- your **physical ability**

- your **willingness** to care for your relative

- whether you are **currently working** or whether you wish to work

- anything else you feel is **relevant to the situation**.

When assessment has been done the care manager will discuss the services that are required for your relative before drawing up a plan of care.

The services that are to be provided should be listed on the care manager's plan of care for your relative. Ask for a copy to be given to you.

Some of the services offered may include:

- provision of equipment (for example, bath hoist)

- help towards installation of a telephone

- respite care

- home adaptations (for example, wheelchair ramps)

- day centre care.

The social worker may ask to do your assessment (the carer's) at the same time as doing the one for your relative. If you prefer a confidential interview however, ask the social worker for a private assessment.

Missing your relative's assessment

If you miss your relative's assessment you will not be able to have a personal assessment until the next review of their care plan. Unless there is a good reason for reassessment, it might not take place for several months or possibly a year.

You can ask for a carer's assessment before the next review if your relative needs reassessing for any reason, perhaps because their condition has deteriorated.

Making the appointment

You will be consulted regarding the time and place of the assessment. This is, of course, flexible in order to suit the people involved.

Before the appointment take time to jot down anything you want to ask or would like taken into account.

Think about:

- how much extra help you need to care for your relative

- whether you need extra equipment, such as bed tables, a bath hoist

- your other commitments (for example, a baby or toddler)

- how much 'off duty' time you need

- your own physical ability

- your own emotional responses to the situation

- how caring for your relative affects your family and your life

- anything in fact, with which you need help or reassurance.

For further details of the Carer's Act and what it means to you, contact the Carer's National Association, the address and telephone number of which is at the end of the book under Useful Addresses.

CASE STUDIES

Eric comes home

Diary entry: Wednesday, 3 July
It is now several weeks since I had my operation for appendicitis, and I feel fit and well. Eric is coming home tomorrow from the residential home where he has been since I went into hospital. Jenny the carer who helped us before is coming back next week when Eric starts going to day care again. For the first two weeks Eric is going to have an extra day at day care so that I get used to the extra work gradually. Our care manager has given us a lot of support since she first came to see us.

Sunday, 7 July
Things are gradually getting back to normal. I had forgotten how tiring it is to have somebody else to care for especially when they need 'looking after'. Still I'm pleased Eric's home again, I have missed him. I didn't get a chance to mark his things before he went into residential care so some of his clothing got lost and will have to be replaced. I'll speak to the care manager about it if they don't turn up. I hope Mum knows I'm looking after Eric like I always promised her I would!

Anne joins the Samaritans

Diary entry: Monday, 16 June
It's two years today since Faith passed away. I've had such a lot of help from the MacMillan nurses and the members of CRUSE that I would like to do something like that to help other people. Our nearest branch is in the next town some miles away. I don't think I could cope with counselling the bereaved as a long-term commitment anyway.

I answered an advert in our local paper asking for volunteers to join the Samaritans. I've been for an interview and have been accepted for training which starts next week. After that I will be interviewed again and told whether I have been accepted as a Samaritan. If they do accept me I will be working in their office, answering the phone and listening to people who need to talk about their problems.

The branch organiser will ask us what hours we are free to help before we are put on the rota. For the first few weeks we continue with our training which is much more practical. The thing I like is that you're never left on your own. I'm looking forward to this new venture.

Grace's carer leaves

Entry from Milly's diary: Tuesday, 9 April
I had to tell Sally, Grace's friend, that I was leaving. She was very upset until I told her I was going to train for my NVQ. She was interested in what I had done and where I was going to work. I explained that I was going to work in a local nursing home. They give practical training and allow you to go to college every week to learn the theory. I told her that I would have to do some set projects and present them to my colleagues.

Sally thought it sounded like a difficult course to undertake especially as I am going to start at Level Two. She wanted to know how I knew about it. I told her that I'd applied to the local college before finding a nursing home which was already involved in the scheme.

She thanked me for telling her and for giving her enough notice to find a replacement.

Hannah is bored

Diary entry: Friday, 27 September
I do most of the food preparation and cooking, the dusting and some of the ironing but I sometimes feel that I am wasting time doing nothing. I think I need something more to stimulate me and provide new interests in my life, but until now I hadn't found anything I really wanted to do. When my friend Julia came the other day, she told me she was applying to do a degree with the Open University. Now that did interest me. I thought that if we both did the same subjects we could study together.

Wednesday, 9 October
We've now got the brochure so Julia came round for coffee today and we decided which courses we would apply for. Then we sent in our applications.

Wednesday, 6 November
I'm very excited because the OU has accepted our applications and we are waiting to start our studies.

DISCUSSION POINTS

1. Do you feel that you as a carer would benefit from any training?

2. Discuss the carers's needs. Have your needs as a carer been addressed?

3. Is there somebody available who the carer can contact:
    (a) in an emergency
    (b) if help, advice or reassurance *etc* is needed?

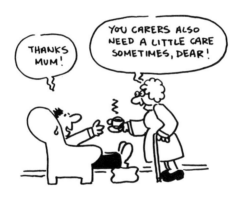

Glossary

Ambulant. Able to walk about from place to place.

Assessing needs. Estimating the amount of care and financial assistance a person requires to enable him or her to live as normal a life as possible.

Back rest. An appliance to support a person when they are sitting up in bed.

Baseline. Normal temperature, pulse *etc* for a particular individual.

Bed cradle. An appliance for relieving the weight of bedclothes on a person in bed.

Care manager. A social worker who assesses care and financial needs of the person needing care to live as normal a life as possible.

Care plan. A detailed ongoing plan of action to ensure a resident's needs/problems are noted and attended to. Care plans are reviewed and updated regularly.

Charitable organisation. An institution set up to provide help to needy people.

Colostomy. A surgically made opening between the colon and the surface of the abdomen which acts as an artificial anus.

Commode. A type of chair that conceals a receptacle which is used as a toilet.

CRUSE. An organisation that helps the bereaved.

DHSS/DSS. Department of Social Security.

Diet. A specific allowance or selection of food. Various diets can be used for different complaints, for example for reducing the weight of someone who is obese.

Domiciliary visit. A visit from the doctor/consultant to a patient's home.

Electric wheelchair. A wheelchair powered by rechargeable batteries.

EN. A trained enrolled nurse.

Exacerbate. An increase in the severity of symptoms.

Fluid balance chart. A record of a persons fluid intake (drinks) and output (urine *etc*).

GP. General practitioner (doctor).

Geriatrician. A doctor who specialises in the diagnosis and treatment of illnesses affecting elderly people.

Grants. One-off or recurrent sums of money given to a person in need.

Helping hand. An appliance used as a hand extension for reaching items.

Jigsaw puzzle folding tray. A tray designed for jigsaw enthusiasts which folds up and protects an unfinished puzzle.

Medication. Drugs given in liquid, tablet or other form to treat a medical condition.

Music and movement. Gentle exercise to music. People with pacemakers should seek medical advice before joining in.

Nausea. A feeling of sickness without actually vomiting.

NVQ. National Vocational Qualification. A training programme combining practical work, lectures, and assessments.

Norton score. A scoring system of assessing a patient's susceptibility to pressure sores.

Occupational therapy. The therapeutic use of crafts or hobbies particularly in the rehabilitation of patients.

Pacemaker. A device fitted to regulate the heart beat.

Parker bath. A specially designed bath allowing easy access for the frail and disabled person. The side is made to rise for entry and is then locked into place whilst the bath is in use.

Prescription. Issued by the doctor for medication. NHS scripts are filled on production of the statutory payment or are free to certain categories of patient. The full cost of private prescriptions has to be born by the patient.

Pressure sore. A sore caused mainly as the result of prolonged local pressure being exerted on the body at various points, for example by blankets or other items causing pressure. Sores can also be caused by prolonged sitting or lying in the same position.

Prognosis. The outcome of an illness or disease.

Prosthesis. Artificial substitute of a missing or damaged part of the body (limbs, dentures, eyes *etc*).

Rehabilitation. Helping a person to regain their former abilities.

Remission. A period of abatement of symptoms in a disease such as multiple sclerosis or leukaemia.

RGN/RN. Registered General Nurse sometimes known as a Registered Nurse.

Spenco mattress. A soft washable mattress used in addition to the usual one to help prevent pressure sores developing.

Syringe driver. A small portable machine used to administer minute dosages of prescribed drugs into the body continuously to give maximum effect. Often used when giving drugs to control severe pain.

Tripod. A walking aid.

Walking frame. A walking aid used by people who can use both arms. Usually known as a Zimmer frame.

Waterlow score. Another method of assessing a patient's susceptibility to pressure sores.

Zimmer frame. A walking frame.

Further Reading

LEAFLETS

Benefits Agency leaflets include:
Which Benefit? FB2
Social Security NI196.
Obtainable from The Benefits Agency Office or by post from HMSO, Oldham Broadway Business Park, Broadgate, Chadderton, Oldham OL9 0JA.
Boots the Chemist produces a leaflet entitled *Do You Look After a Friend or Relative Who is Disabled, Frail or Ill?*
Getting in Right for Carers, Department of Health and Social Security (HMSO, 1991).
Information Needs of Disabled People DSS/18/DHS.
Help the Aged leaflets include:
Bereavement
Can You Claim it?
Claiming Disability Benefits
Healthy Eating
Managing Your Medicines
Questions on Pensions.
A useful National Health Service leaflet is:
HCII Help with Health Costs, from the Department of Health, PO Box 410, Wetherby LS23 7LN.
Stroke: Who Cares? STR/3STR, (Queenspark Market Books).
What next for Carers? COM/169/SO, Social Services Inspectorate, Department of Health.
London Group on Race Aspects of Community Care produces *Black Communities: Who Cares?*

BOOKS

Alzheimer's: A Practical Guide for Carers to Help You Through the Day, Frena Gray Davidson (Piatkus Books, 1995).

Caring for Carers, Christine Ledger (Kingsway Publication, 1992).

Caring for People, Getting it Right for Carers, Department of Health (HMSO, 1991).

Caring for Someone Who Has Had a Stroke, Penny Mares and Philip Coyre (ACE books, 1995).

First Aid Manual (Dorling Kindersley, 1992).

Helping to Care: Handbook for Carers at Home and in Hospital, Betty Kershaw *et al.* (Bailliere, 1989).

The Manual of St John Ambulance, St John Ambulance.

The Parkinson's Disease Handbook, Dr Richard Godwin-Austen.

Practical First Aid, British Red Cross Society (Dorling Kindersley, 1994).

Understanding Nursing Care, Anne Chilman and Meirion Thomas (Churchill Livingstone, 1995).

Useful Addresses

Age Concern England, Astral House, 1268 London Road, Norbury, London SW16 4ER. Tel: (0181) 679 8000.

Arthritis and Rheumatism Council, Copeman House, St Mary's Court, St Mary's Place, Castlefield, Derbyshire S41 7TD. Tel: (0171) 405 8752.

Benefits Agency (Local). See entry in telephone directory.

British Colostomy Association, 113–115 Station Road, Reading, Berkshire RG1 1LG. Tel: (01189) 391537.

British Deaf Association, 38 Victoria Place, Carlisle CA1 1HU. Tel: (01228) 48844.

British Diabetic Association, 10 Queen Anne Street, London W1M 0BD. Tel: (0171) 323 1531.

British Heart Foundation, 14 Fitzhardinge Street, London W1H 4DH. Tel: (0171) 935 0185.

Cancer Support Information, National Support Groups, Cancer Link 46, Pentonville Road, London N1 9BN. Tel: (0171) 833 2451.

Care of the Carers, 143 High Street, Lewes BN7 1XT. Tel: (01273) 476819.

Care of the Dying – British Hospice Information Centre, St Christopher's Hospice, 51–53 Lawrie Park Road, London SE26 6DZ. Tel: (0181) 788 1240.

Carers National Association, 20–25 Glasshouse Yard, London EC1A 4JS. Tel: (0171) 490 8818. Carers line (0171) 490 8898 (Mon–Fri 1pm–4pm).

Citizens' Advice Bureau. Local address and telephone number is listed in the telephone directory.

Counsel and Care for the Aged, Twyman House, Lower Ground Floor, 16 Bonny Street, London NW91 9PG. Tel: (0171) 485 1566.

Crossroads, 10 Regents Place, Rugby, Warwickshire CV21 2PN. Tel: (01788) 833 2451 (for information).

CRUSE (Bereavement Care), Cruse House, 126 Sheen Road, Richmond, Surrey TW9 1UR. Tel: (0181) 940 4818. Helpline (0181) 332 7227 (Mon–Fri 9.30–5pm).

Disabled Living Foundation, 380–384 Harrow Road, London W9 2HU. Tel: (0171) 289 6111.

Help the Aged, St James Walk, Clerkenwell Green, London EC1R 0BE. Tel: (0171) 253 0253. (Help the Aged, Senior Line [Free] (0800) 650065.)

Hi Centre West Kent, Deaf/Hearing Impaired People, 3 Castle Street, Tonbridge, Kent TN9 1BH. Tel: (01732) 773060.

HM Inspector of Anatomy, Department of Health, Wellington House, 133–155 Waterloo Road, London SE1 8UG. Tel: (0171) 273 3776.

Incontinence Advisory Service, 380–384 Harrow Road, London W9 2HU. Tel: (0171) 289 6111 Monday – Thursday.

Jewish Bereavement Counselling Service, 1 Cypres Gardens, London N3 1SP. Tel: (0171) 387 4300 ext 227.

Mobility Trust, 4 Hughes Mews, 143 Chatham Road, London SW1 16H. Tel: (0171) 924 3597.

MS Society of Great Britain, 25 Effie Road, Fulham SW6 1EE. Tel: (0171) 737 6267.

Parkinson's Disease Society, 22 Upper Woburn Place, London WC1H 0RA. Tel: (0171) 383 3513.

Stroke Association, 123–127 White Cross Street, London EC1Y 8JJ. Tel: (0171) 490 7999.

Terence Higgins Trust, 52–54 Gray's Inn Road, London WC1 8JU. Tel: (0171) 831 0330.

The Body Positive, 51B Philbeach Gardens, London SW5 9EB. Tel: (0171) 835 1045.

The Princess Royal Trust for Carers. Tel: (0171) 480 7788.

UK Homecare Association, UKHCA Office, 42 Banstead Road, Carshalton Beeches, Surrey SM5 3NW. Tel: (0181) 288 1551.

Index

CHOOSING A NURSING HOME
How to arrange the right longterm care for an elderly dependant or relative

Mary Webb

Local authorities have recently made severe cutbacks in their budgets for the longterm care of elderly and other people unable to look after themselves at home. This new book meets an urgent need for impartial practical advice on how to plan for the longterm care of an elderly or other dependant relative. It explains how to discuss things with the family, the GP and the local authority, how to shortlist suitable homes, how to overcome emotional difficulties, how to deal with all the financial implications (including those for the family home), how to deal with admission, settling in, visits and a host of other practical details. Mary Webb SRN is an experienced matron/manager who has worked in several nursing homes over the years. She now works for a firm of Nursing Home Management Consultants.

160pp. illus. 1 85703 318 3.

SUCCESSFUL GRANDPARENTING
How to manage family relationships and practical issues

Doris Corti

The average life expectancy is increasing. More people are likely to experience the joys and sorrows of being a grandparent for a longer period of their life. Being a grandparent is different to being a parent. Expectations are different. Many grandparents find that the requirements for bringing up children in today's changing world are very different to what was the norm when they were parents. This new book gives practical advice on such diverse aspect as finances, housing, childminding, taking the role of step-grandparent, sharing grandchildren's upbringing, diplomacy, and obtaining access to children when parents separate or divorce. The answers to these and other problems are given in this book, as well as the names and addresses of helpful organisations. As well as grandparents, typical readers of this book will include grandparents-to-be, retirement groups, library readers, counsellors in church organisations and citizens advice bureaux. Doris Corti has three grandchildren and is an active member of the Grandparents Association.

112pp. illus. 1 85703 307 8.

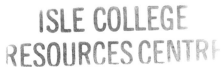

MANAGING YOUR PERSONAL FINANCES
How to achieve financial security and survive the shrinking welfare state

John Claxton

Life for most people has become increasingly beset by financial worries, and meanwhile the once-dependable prop of state help is shrinking. Today's financial world is a veritable jungle full of predators after your money. This book will help you to check your financial health and prepare a strategy towards creating your own welfare state and financial independence. Find out in simple language with many examples and case studies how to avoid debt, how to finance your home, how to prepare for possible incapacity or redundancy and how to finance your retirement, including care in old age. Discover how to acquire new financial skills, increase your income, reduce outgoings, and prepare to survive in a more self-reliant world. John Claxton is a chartered management accountant and chartered secretary; he teaches personal money management in adult education.

160pp. illus. 1 85703 328 0.

DEALING WITH A DEATH IN THE FAMILY
How to manage the practical and emotional difficulties surrounding a death

Sylvia Murphy

Much as we may prefer to avoid thinking about it, sooner or later every family has to face up to the death of one of its members. This book is a must for everyone who has to work their way through the practical maze of legal and social arrangements which must be completed before they can be left in peace to mourn the loved one. It explains what needs to be done at every stage from the realisation of approaching death, to registering the death, arranging an appropriate funeral, obtaining probate for a will and finally being left alone to get on with life. Sylvia Murphy BA MPhil works as an administrator for a bereavement counselling service in a hospice. She has twenty years' experience of writing, administration and teaching and she has recently had to find her own way through the after-death maze several times. She lives in St Austell, Cornwall.

128pp. illus. 1 85703 322 1.

How To Books provide practical help on a large range of topics. They are available through all good bookshops or can be ordered direct from the distributors. Just tick the titles you want and complete the form on the following page.

- Apply to an Industrial Tribunal (£7.99)
- Applying for a Job (£8.99)
- Applying for a United States Visa (£15.99)
- Backpacking Round Europe (£8.99)
- Be a Freelance Journalist (£8.99)
- Be a Freelance Secretary (£8.99)
- Become a Freelance Sales Agent (£9.99)
- Become an Au Pair (£8.99)
- Becoming a Father (£8.99)
- Buy & Run a Shop (£8.99)
- Buy & Run a Small Hotel (£8.99)
- Buying a Personal Computer (£9.99)
- Career Networking (£8.99)
- Career Planning for Women (£8.99)
- Cash from your Computer (£9.99)
- Choosing a Nursing Home (£9.99)
- Choosing a Package Holiday (£8.99)
- Claim State Benefits (£9.99)
- Collecting a Debt (£9.99)
- Communicate at Work (£7.99)
- Conduct Staff Appraisals (£7.99)
- Conducting Effective Interviews (£8.99)
- Coping with Self Assessment (£9.99)
- Copyright & Law for Writers (£8.99)
- Counsel People at Work (£7.99)
- Creating a Twist in the Tale (£8.99)
- Creative Writing (£9.99)
- Critical Thinking for Students (£8.99)
- Dealing with a Death in the Family (£9.99)
- Do Voluntary Work Abroad (£8.99)
- Do Your Own Advertising (£8.99)
- Do Your Own PR (£8.99)
- Doing Business Abroad (£10.99)
- Doing Business on the Internet (£12.99)
- Emigrate (£9.99)
- Employ & Manage Staff (£8.99)
- Find Temporary Work Abroad (£8.99)
- Finding a Job in Canada (£9.99)
- Finding a Job in Computers (£8.99)
- Finding a Job in New Zealand (£9.99)
- Finding a Job with a Future (£8.99)
- Finding Work Overseas (£9.99)
- Freelance DJ-ing (£8.99)
- Freelance Teaching & Tutoring (£9.99)
- Get a Job Abroad (£10.99)
- Get a Job in America (£9.99)
- Get a Job in Australia (£9.99)
- Get a Job in Europe (£9.99)
- Get a Job in France (£9.99)
- Get a Job in Travel & Tourism (£8.99)
- Get into Radio (£8.99)
- Getting into Films & Television (£10.99)

- Getting That Job (£8.99)
- Getting your First Job (£8.99)
- Going to University (£8.99)
- Helping your Child to Read (£8.99)
- How to Study & Learn (£8.99)
- Investing in People (£9.99)
- Investing in Stocks & Shares (£9.99)
- Keep Business Accounts (£7.99)
- Know Your Rights at Work (£8.99)
- Live & Work in America (£9.99)
- Live & Work in Australia (£12.99)
- Live & Work in Germany (£9.99)
- Live & Work in Greece (£9.99)
- Live & Work in Italy (£8.99)
- Live & Work in New Zealand (£9.99)
- Live & Work in Portugal (£9.99)
- Live & Work in the Gulf (£9.99)
- Living & Working in Britain (£8.99)
- Living & Working in China (£9.99)
- Living & Working in Hong Kong (£10.99)
- Living & Working in Israel (£10.99)
- Living & Working in Saudi Arabia (£12.99)
- Living & Working in the Netherlands (£9.99)
- Making a Complaint (£8.99)
- Making a Wedding Speech (£8.99)
- Manage a Sales Team (£8.99)
- Manage an Office (£8.99)
- Manage Computers at Work (£8.99)
- Manage People at Work (£8.99)
- Manage Your Career (£8.99)
- Managing Budgets & Cash Flows (£9.99)
- Managing Meetings (£8.99)
- Managing Your Personal Finances (£8.99)
- Managing Yourself (£8.99)
- Market Yourself (£8.99)
- Master Book-Keeping (£8.99)
- Mastering Business English (£8.99)
- Master GCSE Accounts (£8.99)
- Master Public Speaking (£8.99)
- Migrating to Canada (£12.99)
- Obtaining Visas & Work Permits (£9.99)
- Organising Effective Training (£9.99)
- Pass Exams Without Anxiety (£7.99)
- Passing That Interview (£8.99)
- Plan a Wedding (£7.99)
- Planning Your Gap Year (£8.99)
- Prepare a Business Plan (£8.99)
- Publish a Book (£9.99)
- Publish a Newsletter (£9.99)
- Raise Funds & Sponsorship (£7.99)
- Rent & Buy Property in France (£9.99)
- Rent & Buy Property in Italy (£9.99)

How To Books

___ Research Methods (£8.99)	___ Use the Internet (£9.99)
___ Retire Abroad (£8.99)	___ Winning Consumer Competitions (£8.99)
___ Return to Work (£7.99)	___ Winning Presentations (£8.99)
___ Run a Voluntary Group (£8.99)	___ Work from Home (£8.99)
___ Setting up Home in Florida (£9.99)	___ Work in an Office (£7.99)
___ Spending a Year Abroad (£8.99)	___ Work in Retail (£8.99)
___ Start a Business from Home (£7.99)	___ Work with Dogs (£8.99)
___ Start a New Career (£6.99)	___ Working Abroad (£14.99)
___ Starting to Manage (£8.99)	___ Working as a Holiday Rep (£9.99)
___ Starting to Write (£8.99)	___ Working in Japan (£10.99)
___ Start Word Processing (£8.99)	___ Working in Photography (£8.99)
___ Start Your Own Business (£8.99)	___ Working in the Gulf (£10.99)
___ Study Abroad (£8.99)	___ Working in Hotels & Catering (£9.99)
___ Study & Live in Britain (£7.99)	___ Working on Contract Worldwide (£9.99)
___ Studying at University (£8.99)	___ Working on Cruise Ships (£9.99)
___ Studying for a Degree (£8.99)	___ Write a Press Release (£9.99)
___ Successful Grandparenting (£8.99)	___ Write a Report (£8.99)
___ Successful Mail Order Marketing (£9.99)	___ Write an Assignment (£8.99)
___ Successful Single Parenting (£8.99)	___ Write & Sell Computer Software (£9.99)
___ Survive Divorce (£8.99)	___ Write for Publication (£8.99)
___ Surviving Redundancy (£8.99)	___ Write for Television (£8.99)
___ Taking in Students (£8.99)	___ Writing a CV that Works (£8.99)
___ Taking on Staff (£8.99)	___ Writing a Non Fiction Book (£9.99)
___ Taking Your A-Levels (£8.99)	___ Writing an Essay (£8.99)
___ Teach Abroad (£8.99)	___ Writing & Publishing Poetry (£9.99)
___ Teach Adults (£8.99)	___ Writing & Selling a Novel (£8.99)
___ Teaching Someone to Drive (£8.99)	___ Writing Business Letters (£8.99)
___ Travel Round the World (£8.99)	___ Writing Reviews (£9.99)
___ Understand Finance at Work (£8.99)	___ Writing Your Dissertation (£8.99)
___ Use a Library (£7.99)	

To: Plymbridge Distributors Ltd, Plymbridge House, Estover Road, Plymouth PL6 7PZ. Customer Services Tel: (01752) 202301. Fax: (01752) 202331.

Please send me copies of the titles I have indicated. Please add postage & packing (UK £1, Europe including Eire, £2, World £3 airmail).

☐ I enclose cheque/PO payable to Plymbridge Distributors Ltd for £ ▢

☐ Please charge to my ☐ MasterCard, ☐ Visa, ☐ AMEX card.

Account No. ▢▢▢▢▢▢▢▢▢▢▢▢▢▢

Card Expiry Date ▢ 19 ☎ **Credit Card orders may be faxed or phoned.**

Customer Name (CAPITALS) ....

Address ....

.... Postcode ....

Telephone .... Signature ....

Every effort will be made to despatch your copy as soon as possible but to avoid possible disappointment please allow up to 21 days for despatch time (42 days if overseas). Prices and availability are subject to change without notice.

Code BPA